STRIVE

STRIVE

VENUS WILLIAMS

WITH MYATT MURPHY

8 STEPS TO FIND YOUR AWESOME

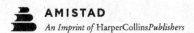
AMISTAD
An Imprint of HarperCollinsPublishers

This book contains advice and information relating to health care. It should be used to supplement rather than replace the advice of your doctor or another trained health professional. If you know or suspect you have a health problem, it is recommended that you seek your physician's advice before embarking on any medical program or treatment. All efforts have been made to assure the accuracy of the information contained in this book as of the date of publication. This publisher and author deny liability for any medical outcomes that may occur as a result of applying the methods suggested in this book.

HarperCollins books may be purchased for educational, business, or sales promotional use. For information, please email the Special Markets Department at SPsales@harpercollins.com.

FIRST EDITION

Designed by Leah Carlson-Stanisic

Smiley face emoji on p. 101 © martialred/Adobe Stock

Library of Congress Cataloging-in-Publication Data has been applied for.

ISBN 978-0-06-327823-3

24 25 26 27 28 LBC 5 4 3 2 1

Dedicated to those whose strive I've always admired,
Oracene, Richard, Serena, Sonya, Isabel, and Althea.
And those who always helped me strive for more,
Isha, Lyndrea, Jorge and Zina, and Reilly.

CONTENTS

STRIVE

BEFORE WE START, I MUST ASK YOU A SERIOUS QUESTION: IF I TOLD YOU THAT LIVING YOUR BEST LIFE POSSIBLE IS ACTUALLY EASY— WOULD YOU BELIEVE ME?

INTRODUCTION

Because here's the thing: I've been asked so many questions throughout my career about every aspect of my life since I was a teenager, and I mean every personal question you can think of. What I eat, how I train, what I do to unwind—believe me, it gets personal sometimes. But the one question I hear most often is, How do you manage to do it all?

Well, guess what? I don't. In fact, some days I can barely manage a couple things, let alone everything I should be handling all at once.

Throughout my entire career, everyone has just naturally assumed I'm some kind of superhuman multitasker who lucked out with great genetics and this desire to run full steam twenty-four seven, and I get that. Most people assume that pro athletes, or, for that matter, anyone who performs at a high level in whatever they do, must be freaks of nature who crush every goal they have for themselves without breaking a sweat and with a smile as they do it. But I'll let you in on something only my family and closest friends know about me.

As regimented as most people *think* I am, my approach to everything in my life—especially when it comes to my health and well-being—is guided by a "shortcut" that keeps me from ever burning out on a lifestyle that I believe in and want to live for the rest of my life.

The truth is anything that I've ever accomplished and any obstacle I've ever overcome, especially the ones that mattered most and made the greatest difference in my life, has come from making the right series of choices that have allowed me to keep one promise to myself:

Make it easy, make it enjoyable, but—most of all—make it exciting.

As an athlete, a businesswoman, and simply a person trying to live her best life possible, I've always striven to keep things manageable, engaging, and fun. It's about creating a path of least resistance for yourself as often as possible, because life is beautiful, but it has its challenges. So why make it more difficult? When I stick with this mindset, no matter what my immediate or long-term goals might be to improve my life, things always fall into place a lot faster with less effort or less stress. Adopting this mindset works without fail while simultaneously providing me with peace of mind every step of the way. See, living your best life possible has nothing to do with luck or winning the DNA lottery. It's all about whether you choose to STRIVE.

Are you ready to STRIVE toward your best life possible? Good, because I'm more than ready to be your guide. Let's do this!

CHAPTER 1

WHAT DOES IT MEAN TO "STRIVE"?

I believe tough love is vital. Why? Because it leads to self-awareness when we show tough love to ourselves. That self-awareness leads to success because only then do we get a true understanding of all of our strengths, weaknesses, and opportunities. But at the same time, I'm a fair person. I don't believe in perfection for a lot of reasons, but the biggest is because trying to be perfect all the time is just not enjoyable whatsoever. I mean, c'mon! People who only eat vegetables and never have an ounce of sugar in their life? That sounds boring, and I don't trust them.

Okay, maybe I'm kidding about that last part, but I mean, who can actually do that? Who has the willpower to resist unhealthy foods all the time without ever having the urge to reach for a comfort food every once in a while? Who can seriously stick with a strict, healthy lifestyle without messing up at some point during the day? I consider myself a pretty strong person, and even I can't do that. And I've had to be on top of what's best for my body from a performance standpoint pretty much all my life.

But when I was diagnosed with Sjögren's syndrome a decade ago, my philosophy was put to its greatest test. Finding out I had an incurable autoimmune disorder—one that flares up unexpectedly, causing pain, numbness, and fatigue—was one of the hardest things to accept, especially when my career expects me to be at my physical best.

Being passionate about health and wellness isn't just a hobby for me. It's something I've researched and explored all my life. That's why I thought I could just push through it with what I already knew. I expected to find some quick fix, a "Band-Aid" that I could place over my Sjögren's and move on. But something prevented me from staying on top of my immune disorder using the same systematic approach I had applied to everything else in my life up until then. And that's when a little sisterly advice to attend a three-week wellness program started me down a path that made me rethink my life.

At the time, I thought I knew all there was to know about health. But it was at the wellness program that I was first introduced to the concept that what you bring to your body—meaning not just what you put *into* it but also what you *apply to* it—ultimately decides how difficult it is for disease to exist within it. I learned that everything we do is interconnected when it comes to our wellness and how when one part isn't working as well as it should, it completely breaks the chain.

This is a concept I already understood through tennis. As an athlete, you not only have to be physically strong but mentally and emotionally strong as well. You can't afford to have any aspect of yourself be in turmoil, because if one is, it's impossible to be your best self at that moment. Turmoil challenges the possibility of long-term success, and even if that success is achieved, you're less likely to enjoy it. To live the healthiest and happiest life possible, you must look at every aspect of yourself—and how each aspect relates to one another.

That three-week program was an eye-opener for me. I immediately stopped looking for the "Band-Aid" and started asking myself: *Why do I even need a Band-Aid in the first place—and can I treat the source of the problem instead of just treating the symptom?* It also made me wonder: *What else don't I understand about health and wellness, and how it's all connected? And is it even* ***possible*** *to bring it all together in a way that is still* ***easy, enjoyable,*** *and* ***exciting?***

With that new perspective, I began seeking out philosophies and strategies both traditional and untraditional within the spaces of health, exercise, rehabilitation, and nutrition. And along the way, I figured out how to combine these different approaches into a road map that lets them work with one another and amplify their individual strengths. This is a strategy that allowed me a decade ago—and still allows me today—to continue doing all the things I love even with Sjögren's, as well as reach any health and wellness goals I ever set for myself.

The STRIVE Solution

It shouldn't be hard to be healthy, and it shouldn't take a lot of work to be well. Every day I commit to eight actions:

- I **observe** everyone and everything around me—including myself.
- I always make time to **appreciate** all that I'm blessed with.
- I accept that my life will never be in **balance**, but I don't stress about that.
- Instead, I throw that energy into things that **enrich** my life and allow me to grow as a person.
- I **soothe** my body and mind by knowing how to slow things down

and put my life on pause, as well as rely on the best therapeutic methods that heal me both externally and from within.

· I understand the power of confidence and make it a practice to **believe** in myself and every step I'm taking along the way.

· I actively look for what **inspires** me and use those little motivations to stay on track and move forward.

· And finally, I always make sure I have at least one goal I'm **striving** toward—something that brings me happiness in its own unique way.

Observe, appreciate, balance, enrich, soothe, believe, inspire, and **STRIVE**. It always comes down to these one-word actions. When you focus on them every day like I do—even for just a few minutes each—these eight tiny but essential actions change your life for the better. I've found that following these eight actions daily is the fastest way to make smarter health decisions turn into habits. Habits that have little choice but to become a simple-to-follow lifestyle over time. And all the hopes you have for yourself in terms of wellness, well—they all fall right into place a lot faster with way less effort or stress.

That is the magic of *STRIVE*. When you do it the way I'm about to show you, feeling happy and accomplished is always within your grasp no matter who you are. Because at the end of the day, if you can truthfully say you did something that honored all eight actions—even if it's the smallest of efforts—then technically, you've won that day. If, before you go to sleep, you can say to yourself . . .

· I **observed** something today.
· I **appreciated** something today.
· I **balanced** something today.
· I **enriched** something today.
· I **soothed** something today.
· I **believed** in something today.

- I **inspired** someone today—either myself or someone else.
- I **strove** toward something today.

. . . if you can do that—and you will, trust me—then that day, you're a success. And, more importantly, you'll be more likely to repeat what you did and to try even more things to capture that proud feeling the very next day—and the next day after that.

Look, I've spent the last decade investing in how to take care of myself because, at the end of the day, it was my responsibility to take care of *me*. Just as it's your responsibility to take care of yourself. Only now, you're not alone. This is the unfailing advice I use every day that makes moving forward with my health and wellness goals easy, enjoyable, and exciting. This is the road map that continues to guide me mentally, physically, and spiritually—not only as an athlete but as a woman, a daughter, a sister, and someone just looking to be happy and healthy for as long as possible.

Simply put, these are the actions that have never failed me.

And now, they are the actions that will never fail you.

CHAPTER 2

THE FOUR TO STRIVE FOR

Now that you know the eight actions you'll be taking each day, let me address the big question I know you're wondering about: *How exactly do you observe, appreciate, balance, enrich, soothe, believe, inspire, and STRIVE?*

There are four significant areas of my life that whenever I've taken a moment to invest in—even when I'm only able to put the slightest bit of energy toward them—always result in payoffs that are well worth the effort.

1. **My diet**
2. **My activities** throughout the day
3. **Who and what's around me**
4. And finally, **myself**

I know what you're thinking. That sounds like a lot of work. I hear you. Overhauling any one of these could easily be a full-time job, let alone all four at the same time! But it really doesn't take much work to see a huge change if you start with these four—it just requires being consistent, giving each a little attention on a regular basis.

I'm serious. Some of the lessons that I'm about to share with you in this book might seem new or profound to you, but many are also super simple and take very little effort or time. That doesn't mean they aren't as game changing. When you think about it, sometimes the simplest things can be the hardest to do because they're so easy to blow off when you're too busy or think you have bigger problems to deal with. But when you have discipline with the smallest of details, you can achieve the biggest of dreams.

Better still, you don't even have to do everything recommended in my book to see incredible results. Honestly, would I love to see you take on as much as you can handle? Well, yeah! Because I'm hard-core and extremely tough on myself, I typically like pushing people toward creating a new standard they can reach for and live up to.

But then again, I don't know what struggles you may have going on in your world. I don't know how many minutes of the day you can give me today versus tomorrow, or what deeply personal and unique goals you've set for yourself. But I do know this—STRIVE works for everyone no matter what your age or activity level may currently be. It's an easy-to-follow program that lets you decide how far you want to take it.

STRIVE Simplified

A lot of lifestyle programs are broken down week by week with incredibly specific instructions when it comes to what they expect you to do. But with STRIVE, here's how it works.

Imagine the Day

What do I mean by that? I'm saying that every morning, you're going to wake up and say these eight actions to yourself:

Observe. Appreciate. Balance. Enrich. Soothe. Believe. Inspire. STRIVE.

I don't care when you do it—whether it's right before you jump out of bed or after you're up and already moving around. But the earlier you say these eight actions to yourself the better, because some of the techniques in this book have a greater impact the sooner you incorporate them into your day.

Why out loud? I mean, do you really have to? Well, I want you to look at it this way. When you say these eight actions aloud, it sets the tone. It reminds you how serious you are about changing your life for the better from minute one of your morning. And the more you say the actions throughout the day, the more often you're reminding yourself that you need to make certain choices to honor these eight actions all day long.

And hey, if you're feeling self-conscious about doing this, then that's the first thing I want you to change. This is *you* we're talking about. This is *your* life and not someone else's. It shouldn't matter what other people think, and if someone has a problem with what you're doing, then explain to them that you're trying to take a serious step toward a better life for yourself. And, if after that, they still think what you're doing is crazy, it might be time to question how supportive that person is and to do something about it. (Don't worry . . . we'll get into what I mean by that a little later.)

Own the Day

From the time you wake up until roughly an hour or two before bedtime, I want you to stay aware of these eight one-word actions, then challenge yourself to figure out a way to apply each action to any of the following areas:

- Your diet
- Your activities
- Who and what's around you
- Yourself

In other words:

1. I want you to **observe** one thing about your diet, activities, who and what's around you, or yourself.
2. I want you to **appreciate** one thing about your diet, activities, who and what's around you, or yourself.
3. I want you to **balance** one thing about your diet, activities, who and what's around you, or yourself.
4. I want you to **enrich** one thing about your diet, activities, who and what's around you, or yourself.
5. I want you to **soothe** one thing with your diet, activities, who and what's around you, or yourself.
6. I want you to **believe** in one thing about your diet, activities, who and what's around you, or yourself.
7. I want you to **inspire** one thing about your diet, activities, who and what's around you, or yourself.
8. Finally, I want you to **STRIVE** toward one thing when it comes to your diet, activities, who and what's around you, or yourself.

How exactly are you going to do that? Easy. Over the next several chapters, I'll show you a variety of fun and creative strategies and methods you can use to apply these eight one-word actions to all areas of your life. Some suggestions are definitely more intense than others, but I am certain you'll find at least one strategy you could try no matter how much time you have or energy you have to give at the start.

Do you have to do them in order each day? Meaning, do you have to observe something before you appreciate something? Do you have to balance something before you enrich something? No, absolutely not, especially when you get going and understand the formula. You can go in any order you wish and do them whenever you want throughout the day.

How should you keep track? Any way you want. In fact, get as creative as you can. Have a notecard in your pocket or purse so that you can check off each action as you complete it. Put each word on a sticky note on your computer and take them down as the day goes on. Add a reminder to your phone that alerts you every hour to perform one of the eight actions. Whatever makes it easiest for you is what I want you to do.

Assess the Day

About an hour or two before bedtime, I want you to ask yourself eight questions:

1. What did I **observe** today?
2. What or who did I **appreciate** today?
3. What did I put into **balance** today?
4. What did I **enrich** today?
5. How did I **soothe** myself (or others) today?
6. What or who did I **believe** in today?
7. What **inspired** me today—or whom did I inspire?
8. What did I **STRIVE** toward today?

Why not right before bedtime? I don't want you to answer these questions right before you go to sleep for good reason. If the day got away from you and you didn't have time to tackle all eight actions (and some days you won't, trust me), this gives you a buffer to take care of whatever actions you missed so you can finish strong. Besides, I don't want you going to sleep feeling guilty that you didn't do everything you could have for the day.

Your only goal is to have an answer for each of those questions. To be able to run through that list and recognize that you affected your life in a positive way using all eight actions that day. And that's it.

Wait, that's it? Seems almost too simple, right?

Perfect, because that's exactly the attitude I want you to have at the beginning of this program. Don't worry, I'll show you a little later how to ramp things up when you need to. Believe me, just because I don't take an extreme approach to achieving health and wellness goals at the start doesn't mean I'm going to be easy on you the whole time. I'm less of a New Age-y type and have a more old-school mindset, if you know what I mean. However, for right now, I just want you to reflect on the eight actions you made that day. Eight things, by the way, that you probably normally wouldn't have done—and that's a perfect place to begin.

The point is, whether you choose to just dip your toe into this book or jump in with both feet, following all eight actions every day makes it far easier to turn smart, healthy choices into lifelong habits without having to overthink them all the time. Collectively, the eight actions create a new standard for you that says, *This is how I choose to live.* And once that happens, you'll forge a healthier lifestyle that you'll always return to because you *want* to—not because you *have* to—and that's when you start winning.

That's the point of STRIVE—to always end every single day feeling like you've won. To feel like you're moving forward because you *are* moving forward, even if that progress for now is accomplished with tiny steps. So long as you stay the course and commit to the program, a little bit is always better than zero.

Are you ready to STRIVE? Then let's explore what makes each of these eight actions so important—and how easy it is to use them collectively to become an even better version of yourself.

CHAPTER 3

OBSERVE

Something my sister Serena has always said about me is that I remain calm under pressure. It's not because I feel or handle stress any differently than everybody else. It's just that I've always been the type to analyze things *first* before I react to anything that deserves attention.

Okay, maybe not *all* of the time—I'm only human, right? But most of the time, whenever I'm faced with a decision (no matter how big or small) or life just comes at me head-on with something it expects me to deal with right then and there, I just step back for a second or two. Instead of feeling like I must react to everything as if it's some sort of crisis, I take time to absorb it all.

Look at it this way: Until you fully understand what you're dealing with, how can you expect to make the right decisions about whatever that is? How can you trust yourself in that moment to pull the right switch when it comes to what's best for you, your family, or anyone around you? Let's face it—you can't. It's just common sense that taking the time to do your homework first when it comes to making any decision about pretty much anything usually pays off. That might not be easy to do in certain circumstances, especially in situations when you may feel you need to act immediately to not miss out. But in most cases, being patient always beats out being impulsive. So why wouldn't you handle your health and wellness in the same way?

In this chapter, I'm going to show you some of the ways I observe my own life from as many angles as possible. I want you to think about the choices you typically make, as well as who and what you regularly surround yourself with. Thoughtfully look inward at yourself. When you have a deeper sense of awareness about your life, that's when you can finally begin making decisions that will stick.

Here's the deal though: For this to really work, I need you to be *honestly aware* right from the start. That's because when it comes to this first action—observe—it is easy to "fudge the facts," if you know what I mean. Often, we don't want to admit our poor habits or to come face-to-face with how far we've slipped from our goals. Sometimes, we don't want to face the negative things that are right in front of us and holding us back because we're ashamed or scared. It's way easier to pretend we don't see these things—or to downplay just how harmful they can be to our overall health.

But remember, STRIVE is a lifestyle that requires pure honesty on your part. Any twisting of the truth doesn't hurt *me*—it only hurts *you*—and anyone else who may be counting on you to improve your health and wellness. Just keep in mind that any observations you'll be making are just for you and no one else. You don't have to share them with anybody if you don't want to. They're just details I want you to acknowledge about yourself to help you dial into what may work best specifically for you and what could be working against you. When you begin changing your life for the better, you'll feel more confident that you're creating healthier habits tailor-made specifically for you.

Observe—The Right Way

To get the most from this first tenet, it's not just about staying silent and being honest. There are still a couple things to know before you start if you want to do it right:

Don't rely on memory. I don't want you just to look around and think you're going to recall everything at the end of the day. I want you to write down or type in any observations you make as you go. And it's entirely up to you how you do it. Send yourself a text or an email. Jot it down on a piece of paper or a Post-it note. But I would recommend that whatever is easiest and draws the least amount of attention is the way to go. If you make it too inconvenient or uncomfortable for yourself, you'll miss out on what makes this action so powerful.

Don't go too crazy. Honestly, once you get going, you're going to see plenty of things about your life that are worth writing down. But trying to cram everything in can sometimes be overwhelming and frustrating. Instead, jot down whatever comes to mind in the moment and don't worry about how many things you have or haven't written down. Just let it flow. So long as every observation is genuinely what you feel in that moment, that's all I care about.

Don't limit yourself. In this chapter, I'm going to want you to observe five areas of your life, but don't let that lock you down into ignoring anything else that may be affecting your life either positively or negatively. There might be portions of your life or decisions that you make that I haven't thought of because, again, it's your life. Just go with whatever presents itself to you that you feel needs to be written down. Just the fact that you *think* something deserves recognition makes whatever that is an important aspect of your life that could need a little more attention either immediately or later.

Finally, don't beat yourself up. After you've written things down, look at everything and ask yourself: Were there times that I felt self-conscious jotting things down? Were there moments when it was easier to keep track and moments when it was more difficult? Did I really write down the most accurate answers—or did I fudge them a little?

If everything went well, then be proud of yourself. And if not, like I said, don't be your worst enemy by punishing yourself for holding back any details. You'll get much better at it as you practice this simple technique. Just take pride in the fact that you're being honest and promise yourself that you'll try better next time.

Observe—Your Diet

It's important to recognize the patterns when it comes to your nutritional habits. You have to own, for better or for worse, what foods you typically reach for, as well as how much and how often you eat—and even why you're eating in the first place.

Having honest awareness of your nutritional habits is the first and most important step if your goal is to change your diet for the better. But this is something many don't bother with because, if you do it the wrong way, that self-assessment can come with a lot of finger pointing and shame. The more mistakes you find with your eating habits, the more down you might be on yourself, leaving you feeling like you should've tried harder or could've done better. But that's not the direction we're trying to go in here.

Let me confess something: I'm definitely not perfect. I'll eat a little bit of everything. But observing how I eat helps me work my way toward building better eating habits.

For example, I'm a late-night eater. I'm not proud of it because I know that isn't always a smart choice to make. But you know what? By observing my diet, I acknowledge that I'm a late-night eater—and I own that about myself. And because I own it, whenever I find myself reaching for foods close to or way past my bedtime, I recognize that bad habit a lot sooner instead of ignoring it, which often makes me less likely to give in to it.

Not because I feel guilty about it but because I own it, I am more aware in the moment that I have a choice to make. I can take a better path. Often, I'll make the right choice. And when I don't, I find that I dwell a little less on it because I know I can make a better choice the next time.

Now it's your turn to own *your* diet. If that sounds daunting, like I'm going to expect you to keep track of every single calorie, don't feel too intimidated. You can save your calculator for later. This is more about recognizing and making yourself accountable for a few eating behaviors. So just do your best to consider integrating any (or as many) of the following observational strategies into your day:

Before You Eat or Drink

Technically, the only time you should be reaching for something to eat or drink is when you're hungry or thirsty. But many other factors could be hiding behind your food choices that have nothing to do with what your body needs nutritionally. So, ask yourself: What behavior is behind this bite? Are you reaching for food or drinks because you're genuinely hungry or thirsty, or could your decision be tied to something else going on?

Are you rewarding yourself for something? I'm not a big believer in consistently treating yourself to food for accomplishing something because it becomes counterproductive. Ultimately, I want you winning as often as possible in all areas of your life. So, if you're in the habit of rewarding yourself with food, the more you win, the more likely you'll be to overeat. That just means that, eventually, you're going to lose when it comes to your overall health.

Are you feeling tired? Reaching for food when you're feeling sluggish during the day can often be a sign of waiting too long between meals or not eating enough. If you're often reaching for food when you're tired, it could be because your blood sugar levels are lower than usual as a result of undereating, which can trigger a craving for food your body can instantly absorb and convert into immediate energy. The problem is that can often mean craving less healthy foods that are rich in simple carbohydrates.

Are you trying to fit in or please someone? How often have you eaten when you're not hungry just because you were someplace where others were probably doing the same? Or felt compelled to taste something simply because someone made it for you? Whatever the case, if you're eating or drinking just because you feel obligated to do so and can't say no, it's important to know how often these types of situations are happening in your life.

Are you feeling rushed or stressed for time? Every day for me is a whirlwind, as I'm sure it is for you too. But if that's how you feel right before you're about to eat, you could be reaching for something less healthy just because it's more convenient.

Are you drinking enough? Often, it's not that we're hungry as much as we're thirsty. Your body is smarter than you may be giving it credit for. When it's dehydrated, it tends to crave foods with high water and sodium content to bring itself more into balance. That can put you at risk of reaching for processed foods that contain a lot of carbohydrates and salt, when all you really need is a little more water during the day.

Are you hoping to recapture a certain memory or feeling? Food is a trigger that a lot of us use to remind ourselves about the past, especially if it's attached to a good memory. I know I have my fair share of snacks that remind me of when I was a kid. But if you're turning to memory triggers too often with foods that aren't as healthy for you, that's something to pay attention to.

Are you trying to hide how you really feel? We call them comfort foods for a reason, right? Whether we're stressed out, depressed, or bored, it's sometimes easier to reach for something to eat or drink instead of getting off our butts and doing something or facing how we feel in the moment. But it's important to address and keep track of how often you use food as an impulsive distraction away from what's really on your mind.

Are you strapped for cash? Most people think that eating healthier costs more, and it can in some instances, but if you're grabbing certain unhealthy foods more often because they're cheaper, that's good to recognize—and plan around—for later.

Are your clothes a little sweaty? In other words, did you just finish exercising, playing a sport, finishing yard work, or doing some form of aerobic activity? These are moments when you really can't blame your body for craving a few more calories.

After You Eat or Drink

Focus on how you feel: I used to love steak. I'm talking I could literally eat steak every day. Back in the day, I lived by the motto "Give me a ribeye or give me death." But only after going to the three-week health seminar with my mom and sister did I first start to really listen to what my body was trying to tell me after eating.

When we got there, we were told that the only thing we were going to be allowed to eat for three straight weeks was raw vegetables. Three. Straight. Weeks. I mean no exceptions. No sneaking in takeout or ordering off-the-menu room service. So, once we heard that, my sister turned to me and said, "We're going out right now and getting a steak and some dessert—because it's our last meal!"

I couldn't help but notice how heavy my stomach felt and how lethargic I was afterward. I literally felt weighed down, which was exactly the opposite of how I felt during the time we started eating a plant-based diet. We complained a little because we felt lighter. "I don't want to feel light!" we all joked, but it was true.

In that case, my observations about how steak affected me were extreme. Your own observations may not be, but what you take in is *always* affecting you either positively or negatively, even if the reaction is slight and hard to notice. That's why, after every meal or snack, you should really sit with yourself and see if you feel better or worse than you did before you started eating or drinking, both physically and mentally.

Even people who journal about **what** they eat often forget to write down how they **feel** after they eat. They never notice whether they feel better or worse, more energetic or sluggish, happier or sadder, proud or disappointed. The answers should always be that you feel better both physically and emotionally about yourself, but if that's not the case with certain meals, you need to acknowledge how often that's happening.

Remind yourself of ratios: Unhealthy foods don't magically show up in my fridge, in my pantry, or on my plate. I'm the one who's guilty of putting them there—and so are you. And you really don't need to be a dietitian to understand the difference between what's healthy and what's junk, do you? Most of us have a general sense of how often we're eating the healthy stuff or sneaking in the crap.

I'm not asking you to write anything down, but instead, do a sort of "off-the-cuff audit" to see which way the pendulum swings between good and bad with every meal. For example, was it pretty much all natural or was it processed food? Is it something you know you should be eating more of, or is it something you honestly know you should be eating less of?

You can do this audit with every meal, or take it a step further and look through your pantry and fridge. Start from the top going to the bottom and just roughly count how many healthy foods you have access to versus unhealthy things.

Take note of the time: Why did you eat or drink at that exact moment? Was it because it was noon and you felt you "needed" to have lunch even though you weren't hungry? Was it later than you usually eat because the day got away from you? Was it a few hours after the last time you had something to eat—or much sooner than that?

Observe—Your Activities

I believe in brutal honesty, especially when it comes to myself and exercise. It's the only way I move forward as a performance athlete, because when I'm not honest, I'm never able to get to my goal.

Having said that, I know this might not be something you want to hear, but it's necessary to come right out and say it: If you're not satisfied with where you're at physically—whether that pertains to your current weight, your shape, your performance, your energy level, your overall health, or all of the above—you're most likely not doing enough in terms of being active. You might even genuinely believe you're putting in more effort than you actually are. But the good news is you can decide to do something about it and change all that about yourself. The truth is just where you are right now—but it's not where you have to stay.

Now, I don't know how active you are on a regular basis, and you might not even know yourself, but you're about to have a better sense. That's why I want you to observe all your activities. What do I mean by activities? I mean anything that gets your heart beating a little faster, whether that's exercise, participating in a sport, your job (if it's a physical one), or even doing chores or tasks around the house. But first, let's start with the obvious one, which is how far you walk each day.

Observe your steps. It's important to know how much you're moving around versus sitting or standing around. You can use the step counter on your phone, but if you're not the type to have your phone on you twenty-four seven (if that is you, I'm impressed), then buying a simple pedometer will do. Whichever method you choose, I have a few ground rules you absolutely must follow:

No peeking. I don't want you to observe how much you're walking *during* the day because being curious might make you walk a little more than you typically would after seeing that number. Just let your phone do its thing and wait until the very end of the day to check it.

No weekends. For most of us, Saturday and Sunday are the two days when we either play catch-up and try to do a million things at once, or we sit around to relax from a long week and do nothing at all. But Mondays through Fridays are typically routine and are great days to judge just how much you truly move on an average basis.

Observe what's holding you back. When I say, "holding you back," I mean anything that might be preventing you from exercising beyond the typical "I don't have any time" excuse most people turn to. No, I mean really look at the fringe things that may not seem important but could be keeping you from investing in exercise with whatever time you do have. For example:

Do you feel comfortable in your workout gear? It's so important to feel good and not self-conscious about not just what you wear but about how you feel in it. That said, consider whether the reason you're not as active is because you don't feel comfortable wearing workout attire or showing too much of your body. Or maybe your clothes are too constrictive and don't let you move freely. Or could you be feeling self-conscious because the wardrobe you have isn't quite fancy enough for the gym you choose to work out in. Wearing something you feel good in can make the difference in whether you give it your all that day or hold yourself back from getting moving in the first place.

Do you have access to exercise equipment? You really don't need much to challenge your muscles and rev up your metabolism. In fact, the workout I'll suggest later will prove that point. But if this is your biggest problem, know that you don't need the latest and greatest exercise equipment to get the job done.

Do you need others around you? I can't play tennis without having somebody across the court, so could it be that you need more people to sweat it out with to do the activity you'd prefer? Or even if it's a certain activity you could do alone, is the fact that you want a walking partner or an exercise buddy instead of being by yourself preventing you from trying as hard as you could be?

Observe your exercise habits. The moments before, during, and after exercise ultimately decide whether you're wasting your time or truly working toward your fitness and health goals. That's why it's key to observe yourself before, during, and after you work out to answer each of the questions in this section truthfully.

Before You Exercise . . .

Do you have a game plan? It might be fun to fly by the seat of your pants when it comes to exercise, but it's not doing your body any favors if you're doing that every single time. No matter what your fitness goals may be, you should have some sort of program in place that's designed to help you achieve them.

Is this the smartest time to do it? Look at the rest of your day and assure yourself that whatever block of time you put aside to be active was the wisest—at least most of the time. If not, then you could be unknowingly rushing through your workouts, trying to pull them off when you're too tired, or interfering with performing at your best as often as possible.

Are you ready to give it your all? There are some people who love to exercise, and then there's the majority of us. The ones that do it because we have to, not necessarily because we want to. Hey, I'm not judging if that's you, because you're far from alone. But just because you're not overly enthusiastic about exercise, that's no reason not to bring your A game. What your mindset is *before* you're active determines how much you put into that activity, so you need to be ready to bring it.

As You Exercise . . .

Are you tracking your rest time? How long you rest between resistance-training exercises matters. Limiting that time to thirty seconds or less doesn't give your muscles enough time to recover and makes it more difficult to maintain strength, but it's great for building muscular endurance. Waiting two minutes or more between exercises helps them fully restore their strength but doesn't work on muscular endurance. You should always have some sense of how long you're waiting in between movements.

Are you pushing yourself enough? Exercising can be fun, but if it feels too easy, then odds are you're not challenging your body hard enough to make much progress. Achieving your fitness goals isn't just about putting in the time. It's about putting in the effort. If you're able to carry on a full conversation with someone as you exercise without ever needing to catch your breath, you're probably working out at a level that's below where you should be. That's where the Rate of Perceived Exertion (RPE) Scale comes in.

As you exercise, rank how hard you're pushing yourself on a Rate of Perceived Exertion Scale of 0 to 10 as follows:

- 0: Standing still and doing nothing.
- 1 to 2: A slow tempo where having a conversation isn't a problem.
- 3 to 4: A light tempo that lets you talk comfortably with minimum effort.
- 5 to 6: A medium-fast tempo you could talk through but couldn't sing through.
- 7 to 8: A high-intensity tempo that makes it difficult to do anything but speak in short phrases.
- 9 to 10: A seriously high-intensity tempo that makes it impossible to speak.

Are you pushing yourself too hard? Some people take the approach that if a little of something is good for them, then a lot is even better. Exercise doesn't always work that way, and when we're trying things that are too difficult for us, we sort of know it, right? Be honest with yourself about any movements, exercises, or activities that may be beyond your body's capabilities—for now at least.

After You Exercise . . .
Did anything interrupt your focus? Think about anything that might have distracted you during your workout. Maybe it was the music? Was it too crowded? Did the friend you brought along talk too much and not take the workout seriously? Once you're aware of what's interfering with your exercise, think of a way to change that outcome the next time.

Do you feel proud? Because you should. I'm not saying you have to set a record every time you're exercising, but personal pride can come from just knowing that you accomplished what you set out to do. But if you're walking out of the gym or away from an activity feeling down on yourself, try to figure out why. So long as you tried your best, you should always feel proud of yourself.

Observe—Who and What's Around You

Sometimes part of the struggle with trying to live a healthier lifestyle isn't entirely our fault. The things we surround ourselves with play a huge role in whether we succeed or fail, and whether we're effortlessly swimming with the tide or fighting furiously against it.

So how do you create an environment that supports you? How do you surround yourself with the right things to keep you on track and less likely to stray? It takes a 360° look at the places where you make your most important choices—the choices that ultimately decide which direction your life will go.

It also takes a village to be victorious, and who you choose to bring into your life makes certain healthy decisions easier, harder, or even impossible to execute. But this is where it gets tricky because each of us has our own network. But that doesn't mean there aren't a few traits you can observe regarding those around you and how you feel and act around them.

You see, no matter how great or how small of a presence someone is in your life, every single relationship is an investment. It's an investment of time that you're putting toward someone else and that they're putting into you. An investment that should always be growing and working *for* you instead of *against* you, which is why it's so critical to pull people into your life who nurture it instead of take from it.

So, are you getting the best return on your investments? And equally important, are you bringing value into the lives of those around you as well? The only way to find out means taking an honest look at those in your life, especially if your plan is to have it be your best life possible.

Observe the level of everyone's glass. Optimism and pessimism are infectious. Hang around a glass-half-full type of person who always finds the bright side of everything, and your glass will have a little more in it by default. But it works both ways. Spend too much time with a glass-half-empty type who's always complaining, and it pokes a hole in the bottom of yours just as quickly.

For now, just gauge everyone's glass and take a tally of the optimists and pessimists in your inner circle and outer circles—anyone you find you're either spending at least a few minutes talking to or having to listen to. That percentage (whichever way it leans) basically indicates the amount of positive or negative vibes you're absorbing daily.

Observe who makes you beam. Every time you're around someone you encounter on a regular basis, question whether they genuinely make you happy.

Look, not everybody you meet, work with, live with, or spend time with is going to light up your world every second of the day. That's just not realistic. Plus, there are different levels of happy, right? You have people who instantly make you smile the moment you see them, or even when you're just thinking about them. Then there are others who may not have that same sort of impact, but you're still happy to see them.

I'm not asking you to rate anyone from a scale of 1 to 10. Instead, just leave it as a yes or no, just so you have a better idea of how many people within your world make you smile.

Observe who lets you be you. We're never our truest selves with most people because we can't always be. That's not a bad thing—it's just what it is. Can you imagine if everyone ran around and acted like their real selves at their job, at church, or in public? Trust me, it wouldn't be pretty.

But everybody needs at least one person who gets them, because when you have that presence in your life, it gives you that shot of confidence you might really need in moments when you have self-doubt. They remind us that we are worthy during times when we are too harsh on ourselves. They remind us that someone likes us, even when we think we're too difficult or unlikable.

Observe who you mirror. We may not always see it in ourselves, but what others do and how they act around us can cause us to do the exact same things and act the exact same way, either consciously or unconsciously. That's why, as you scan those around you, see if you can spot habits, actions, behaviors, or anything— either good or bad—that you find yourself doing either around them or when they're not around (but because of them). Some easier connections to notice could include:

- If you're dining with them, are your eating habits your own, or are you imitating theirs?
- When you're exercising, do you follow a routine that's best for you, or just go with the flow with whatever others are doing?
- If they seem stressed, do you become stressed?
- When they complain, do you find yourself complaining?
- If they start bragging about their weekend, do you feel you have to do the same?

Observe who helps you grow. Look, not everybody in your life is going to have a huge positive effect on you. But any person you let into your world should be helping you move forward, even if it's just a little bit.

When you open your eyes a little wider, it's obvious to see who falls into this category. They are usually the ones who, when things aren't going right with you, ask how they may help instead of just inserting themselves into the conversation by telling you how bad they have it. They're the people who, when you're uncertain about a decision, help you work through it or suggest a variety of options to try. Basically, when you're going through hell, they're either by your side or the first to check in—instead of just checking out.

However, these people don't have to be close friends who always have your back. They may not even know you on a personal level (like a teacher or mentor, for example). Anyone who educates, inspires, and/or supports you in some way—even if they're not aware of their empowering impact on you—still counts in my book.

Observe where you eat. Are you sitting at a dining table, or is the dining table your desk? Are you always eating at home or forever eating out? Do you prefer the kitchen counter or the front seat of your car? Where you eat most frequently dictates what options you have when it comes to eating. But that's not the only thing I want you to observe:

Is your kitchen cluttered? If so, you could be making it less convenient to prepare healthier meals, which means you're more likely to rely on prepackaged and other unhealthy foods that tend to be more convenient.

Are you more often with others or alone when you eat? We may make bad choices or binge when we're flying solo, whether out of boredom or because no witnesses are around to call us out.

But sometimes, we might find ourselves throwing back unnecessary calories when around friends to fit in or because food is being pushed on us. Observing who you dine with most often—others or yourself—may give you a better idea about whether the company you keep is negatively impacting your diet.

What's directly in front of you? If it's a TV, a computer screen, your phone, or anything that's capturing your attention more than the food on your plate, you could be mindlessly tossing back food you don't need and/or not as focused on your food choices.

Observe what places change you. When I say "change you," I'm talking about your mood. I want you to observe if any places make you feel different from how you normally feel, for better or for worse.

It's so funny how the answers can be so different depending on who I ask. Some people will tell me how their job is a major drag, while others light up about their nine-to-five gig because that's where they feel most appreciated. I know people who love being around others, and also people who prefer time to themselves. Some love the craziness of city life, while others crave the fresh air of a local park.

That's why I want you to observe all the places you frequent most often—work, home, locations while running errands, kids' events, the gym, the homes of friends or extended family, etc.—and look for any changes in your mood. If certain places are pulling you down, it's important to acknowledge them to figure out what you might do to change how you feel, to spend less time there, or to avoid that place all together.

Observe what surrounds you. Stop reading right now (actually, wait until you finish this sentence) and take in a 360° view around you. I mean look at everything not bolted down—and even what might be bolted down! The pictures on your table, the view from your window, even the paint on your walls. Observe all the things constantly present in your life from morning until night—at home, your job, wherever—and ask:

Does it bring me up or down? I'm not expecting you to figure out whether your stapler or microwave is making you depressed. In fact, most of the things you'll observe probably won't make you feel one way or the other. But pay attention to anything that does change your mood—even in the slightest—and acknowledge that.

Does it make me anxious or proud? Maybe it's frustrating for you to see that hole in the wall you've been meaning to fix or that to-do list that's collecting dust. Or you beam whenever you walk past that award you got or that picture your kids drew for you. There are always little triggers around us that consciously or unconsciously affect our stress levels.

Finally, can I do something about it? Meaning, if something is preventing you from being happier or healthier, can you get rid of it or make it less noticeable? And if the opposite is the case, and something is encouraging and supportive, can you pick a better spot for it so that you see it more often, or can you find other things just like it that make you feel the same way?

Observe where you call it a night. Before you go to bed, consider how your environment could potentially influence your sleep. Even the teeniest of distractions can sometimes secretly overstimulate your brain, making it a little more difficult to fall asleep, or worse, robbing you from getting a deeper, sounder sleep through the night. Here are just a few things to observe:

Are your other senses equally satisfied? Usually, the two major concerns are whether it's too noisy or too bright to sleep, but pay attention to and observe how your other senses may be affected as well. Does the room have a certain scent to it that affects you in any way? Is the bed, as well as whatever you're wearing to it, comfortable? Observe anything and everything that is triggering your senses one way or the other.

How close are any potential distractions? This could be your phone, the alarm clock, the remote control, that book you can't put down, the folder of work you took home, your partner who fidgets too much or snores. Some sleep disturbers are painfully obvious, while others may not necessarily be as noticeable. Pay attention to all the things in your bedroom that could be adding up in a way that's stealing your quality of sleep.

What's going on with your belly? Did you just eat something? Drink something? Is your stomach grumbling or is it full? For now, just keep a close eye on your eating and drinking habits before bedtime and anything that could be making it more difficult to sleep.

Observe—Yourself

Welcome to what might be (for some) the second-hardest portion of this book—the "appreciating yourself" portion being the number-one hardest section, which I'll talk about later.

I say this because, even though no one is with us more than ourselves, often we are the last person to truly observe ourselves for who we really are. Because when you don't try to look at yourself and the life you're leading, you never have to come face-to-face with whatever's in your life that you might not want to address.

But not looking at yourself closely is called avoidance, and if you're really in this game to change your life for the better, you'll go absolutely nowhere until you finally acknowledge that person in the mirror.

So, what is the life you want? Can you see it? Because if you can, you must know that you can't change your situation—you can't create that life for yourself—until you change your attitude toward being afraid of what you might find as you pick yourself apart. The only way you're going to have the best chance of rebuilding a better you is if you have a positive attitude toward breaking yourself down—so let's begin.

Observe yourself from head to toe. Chances are you've probably done this one thousand times already while stepping out of the shower, standing in your closet wondering why certain clothes don't fit, or looking at someone else's body and then down at your own. But that's just it. I don't want you comparing yourself to anyone else. That's definitely not the point of this exercise. In fact, I want you to imagine that you're one of a kind, because you are.

I'm not being all spiritual when I say that—I'm saying it because it's fact. Everything about you from head to toe is what makes you, well, you. All I want you to do is look at yourself objectively, not judgmentally, and make yourself aware of all the parts that technically total up to you.

However, I don't want your observations to stop at your appearance. Living the best life possible is also about paying attention to how you feel. That's why I also want you to give yourself an "all-access audit" for anything out of the ordinary. For example:

· Are there any specific places on your body that are achy or sore? Is it chronic or only at certain times?
· When you woke up, were you still sleepy or did you feel refreshed? Did you feel sorer in certain areas, such as your back, legs, or neck,

than when you fell asleep because of how you might have been
positioned?

- Are there certain times of the day when you feel better or worse?
  More tired or more energized?
- Try comparing one arm to your other arm to detect any
  differences in how they feel. You can do the same comparison
  with your legs, each finger and toe, your elbows and knees,
  or any place on your body where you have more than one of
  something.

Observe how you divide your day. We all think differently and
manage our time in different ways. We all have unique tasks, goals,
and obstacles we feel we need to accomplish or overcome or could
pass on for now. That's why managing our time is one of the most
important things we can do for ourselves—but it's also one of the
biggest areas we can easily fail in.

When you assume you don't have enough minutes in your day
to get things done, it becomes that much easier to make excuses
to not do a thing. But I think the big reason most people feel they
don't have time to improve their lives for the better is that they re-
ally don't have the greatest sense of how they're honestly breaking
up their day.

The truth is you have time. We all have time, no matter how
busy we think we are. It's just that a certain portion of your day is
spent pouring minutes into trivial things that don't really matter
or make much of a difference. That's why I want you to observe
your actions for the day (from the time you wake up until you go
to sleep) and break up how you spend it.

You don't have to go minute by minute. Just block it out by the
half hour. (Although to be fair, the more precise you are, the more
accurate a picture you're going to paint for yourself.) For each
block of time, I want you to give it a label: Is it important or un-
important? Is it healthy or unhealthy? That's all I want you to do.

Then the next day, just step back from the breakdown and soak in where your time typically flows.

Observe how far you've come. I don't care if you've never tried a lifestyle program before, put any thought into your diet, exercised a day in your life, or given any consideration to improving your health—everyone starts from somewhere. And that place is rarely zero.

Even if you feel you're at rock bottom with every single aspect of your life, I guarantee you that you're not, because that's impossible. So, when I say, "Observe how far you've come," I mean look at your life and reflect on any areas that you've ever made progress with.

It doesn't have to be anything health related. I'm talking about any aspect of your life, whether that's work, a hobby, school, a skill, being a parent or friend, a specific task or chore, anything that you can technically observe and honestly say to yourself, "You know what? I'm definitely a little bit better at that right now than I was back then."

Seriously, pull it back as far as you want. Take it all the way back to when you were a kid if necessary. Because the point of this observation is to remind yourself that, at one time, you might not have been as good at something, but you grew to become better at it. That sense of gratification and accomplishment you feel about those things is equally possible with any of the changes that I'm going to suggest—trust me. Just remember that.

Observe your thoughts. Oftentimes we're not quite sure why we might be in a certain mood (whether happy, sad, indifferent, etc.), have a little less—or even a little more—motivation than usual, or simply feel a particular way at any given moment. But the answer is available to us, if we take the time to, well, listen to ourselves.

What's playing in the back of our minds—the moments we have with ourselves and things we're thinking about—has such a strong influence on deciding which path we find ourselves on. Your thoughts, no matter what they might be, are affecting you in ways you may not even be aware of—emotionally, physically, spiritually, and mentally. That's why it's vital that you observe what you're thinking about in the moment at every opportunity, and question whether those thoughts are affecting you in either a positive or negative way.

I'm not asking you to psychoanalyze yourself, but instead, take a few seconds to shut the rest of the world out; focus on whatever topic, concern, or thought is playing itself out in your brain; and just pay close attention to how it's making you feel. Is it something you wish you could forget or something you want to hold on to in your head? Is it something that's making you smile, or is it something that's leaving you sad or stressed? Whatever it is, it's important to have better awareness about where your mind wanders and if it's often a place that's more positive than negative (or vice versa).

Observe if you're really invested. How do you feel right at this moment? Are you taking it seriously—or just going through the motions? Because here's the thing: if you're just here to say you showed up, then you're not going to get the most from life, let alone this book.

Will there be weeks when you might be less energetic? Could there be days when you're less motivated to follow this program than others? If I ask you this question several times throughout the day, will your answer change depending on your mood? Yes, to all the above. But I need your head to be in the game as often as possible for this to work. Because when it's not, I can personally guarantee you'll put less effort into what you need to do for yourself and will be more likely to ignore (instead of acknowledging) what deserved more of your effort and attention. That's why if you only observe one thing about yourself, then make it this—because it sets the tone for everything else.

So, ask yourself: "Am I really invested? Am I ready to put in the work, even if it takes more sacrifice than I may be willing to make or more time than I feel I have to give? Ask yourself this every chance you can. Because on those days when the answer is yes— that's when you'll notice the most results.

CHAPTER 4

APPRECIATE

Once, I was playing in a quarterfinal match at the US Open, and throughout the entire match, all I was thinking was, "Gosh, I'm playing so horribly—what a disaster!" I had won the first set, and I was up in the second set, but I inevitably lost. It wasn't until a few years later that I looked back and realized, "I was up 6–2, 3–1 . . . why did I think that was horrible? I was killing it!" But at the time, I couldn't appreciate anything I was doing, and that mindset ruined the rest of the match for me.

After that, I learned that you must acclimate yourself to remembering how important it is to be appreciative as often as possible. Even if you're having a moment when you want more but you're not reaping the rewards. Even if you want to be better, but you're not quite there yet. Even if you want to pull off perfection, but you're far from perfect—you must appreciate what *you're achieving in the moment*, how much better you've become since you started, and how many "moments of perfection" you've experienced among your mistakes if you want to get to the next level. While it's important to strive to be your best, it's also just as important to see yourself in a way that's positive when you're not quite at your best. Don't get me wrong. Recognize your mistakes when they happen because brutal honesty is important, but you also need to see the great things you're doing to pump yourself up, even if it's the smallest of things.

I grew up as a Jehovah's Witness, and the Bible says, "Let your yes mean yes, and your no mean no"—and my mom was a stickler for that. She would always tell me, "If you say yes to something, then you keep your word. And if you said no, remember that your 'no' is okay too. But whatever you say—you mean it." So I grew up with this strong conviction of always staying true with not just what I say but also what I believe and who I am.

I've always tried to remain grateful for any successes—big and small—that I've been blessed with, both on and off the court. And even when I've experienced criticism along the way, ranging about everything from the shape of my body to my aggressive playing style, I've never changed anything based on others' opinions. Instead, I've always tried to embrace what has set me apart from the pack. Now it's your turn to do the same.

For many people, appreciating where you are can be a hard thing to do. But even if you think you're not succeeding at something, there are always a lot of "little wins" all around you if you look hard enough or make the effort to see them. I don't care how many times you think you've failed trying to lead a healthy lifestyle. We all have a few healthy habits already in place, even if you think you're the furthest from healthy out there.

It's important to slow down long enough to take in those small victories we're knocking out during the day. We become so obsessed with the next plate we think we need to spin that we don't look around and notice the ones we already have effortlessly up in the air. These are the healthy habits we've already accomplished or have locked in place and made routine. But they *are* there, and trust me, you must recognize them because there is a power in appreciating what's already in place in your life from a health and wellness perspective.

If you appreciate at least one thing every day, it makes it easier to embrace and/or pull off other healthy habits later—even habits you might have always struggled with in the past—for a variety of reasons.

When you allow yourself to see how you've already succeeded with your lifestyle, it can help reduce anxiety, depression, stress, and negativity, so you feel better about yourself all day long and sleep better at night. It helps you see the support that's already in place around you, so you know who you can lean on or go to during the tougher times you may have along the way. It also makes you recognize what you're capable of and boosts your self-confidence, which can lead to smarter, healthier choices down the road. Finally, just by having more clarity in what's already present in your life, you may even find yourself less likely to turn to certain negative lifestyle habits you may be falling back on because you let yourself always feel defeated by not recognizing your accomplishments.

But that doesn't mean I want you to appreciate only your achievements. I want you to appreciate your failures as well. Life is a process and it's never a straight path onward and upward. Trust me—I know a little bit about winning or losing. But it's how you react to any challenges, mistakes, and pitfalls that **will**—not **might**—but **will** happen along your health and wellness journey that decides how far you fall backward and how high you fly. You will always have plenty of moments when you struggle to do the right thing, and it's so important to realize that "ups and downs" and "highs and lows" are all part of the game. That's why some of the things you'll be asked to appreciate in this chapter might surprise you. But it's all about knowing how to appreciate those moments when they do so you can learn from them and strive forward.

Appreciate—The Right Way

There are three things I want you to reflect on whenever you're appreciating any aspect of your life:

What makes you feel happy or proud for the right reasons? What I mean by that is this: Some of your talents or accomplishments might impress someone else, but what do you appreciate that brings *you* pride or happiness?

For example, if you already exercise a fair amount each week, but you do it because you like the attention it gets you from others at the gym, then that would be the wrong reason. The things we appreciate shouldn't be to please others or get their approval, but instead should be things we appreciate regardless of what others think.

Which positive choices or healthy activities are in your life because of you and you alone? Strange question, right? I want you to ask yourself this though, because if you have any that you can name, you already have proof that you're capable of pulling positivity into your world. It's a reminder that, at some point, you recognized how important that thing or decision was toward leading a healthier lifestyle, then you stuck to your guns and kept it in your life.

Maybe you already incorporate a lot of vegetables into your diet or get plenty of sleep. Maybe you're already on top of staying active or making smart decisions that keep your blood pressure under control. Whatever healthy choices you're already making, I need you to remind yourself they are in place because of you. Each one is an example of what you're capable of—period.

Is there a way to build on some of your current healthy habits? Just because you recognize and appreciate a positive thing about your life doesn't mean you shouldn't consider how to make that "great" thing even greater. Think about if there's any way to amplify each habit.

For example, if you recognize that a good friend has your back and is encouraging of you leading a healthier lifestyle, ask yourself what you could do to build on that friendship and make it even stronger. If you're proud that you already make smart choices when eating out, ask yourself if there's any way you could make even smarter choices to take it a step further.

Look, if you can't think of ways to do this when first starting the program, that's fine—and don't worry, because you're going to learn lots of tricks and techniques as we go. I just want you to begin thinking this way, because if you can make it second nature to imagine how to improve healthier habits you already have in place, you can take your lifestyle to another level with less effort. It's like adding on to a structure that already has a solid foundation.

When we're continually hustling, we may *feel* we're getting a lot done, but we're not filling ourselves up emotionally and spiritually. We get so distracted by constantly racing toward the next goal or thing that we're less available to the people around us.

Yet when we're productive in a way where we're not only doing what God has called us to do but we're also present in the moment, it raises us emotionally and spiritually. It grants us pause to appreciate those around us and gives us the breather needed to look more closely at what it is we're so desperate to obtain. If you just take a second, you may discover that what you seek is to feel loved—and that love is all around you—but you're running right past it.

Appreciate—Your Diet

Now that you've observed your diet, it's time to give you credit for what you're already naturally doing. It's time to praise when you did something right. But when it comes to what you did wrong, I don't want you spending a second on any mistakes whatsoever.

I mean that. This action is all about appreciation, not criticism and beating yourself up over what you did or didn't do. It's about patting yourself on the back for what you *did*—or at least *tried* to—accomplish with your diet. Even if you didn't do it perfectly, and even if you did it by mistake.

But appreciating what you're getting right doesn't have to be the only thing you could acknowledge about your diet. You can also spend more time appreciating certain aspects about the healthy foods that you're eating, or even how you're eating them. With that in mind, here are some ways you could check off "appreciate" for the day when it comes to your nutritional habits.

Appreciate the healthy stuff you already eat. Pick up any diet book and it's hard not to feel guilty being told what you shouldn't eat because it's bad for you. But I don't care who you are, even the worst eaters can have a few healthy habits occasionally—and that's so important to acknowledge. You need to appreciate what good habits you already have as you start improving your bad habits.

First, appreciation reminds you what you're capable of. I've had so many of my friends give up trying to eat better because they didn't think they had it in them to change. But when you take time every day to appreciate any healthy nutritional habits you already do, you're literally giving yourself proof that you're stronger than you give yourself credit for.

Second, it also shows you that you're not starting from zero. When you feel like you're starting at the bottom, that can sometimes be demoralizing enough to make you give up before you even begin. But we also have areas in our lives where we're already succeeding, just as we all have areas in our lives where we want to be better. By giving yourself credit for the good things you already did, you not only motivate yourself but you regularly remind yourself that you're not as far from your goals as you may think, because you already have a few things in place. In a sense, you bring yourself a little closer to the finish line by moving the starting blocks.

Appreciate every nutrient. Every healthy food has at least *one* thing inside it that's doing your body good. Maybe that's the reason you ate it in the first place, sort of like when you reach for an orange if you're feeling sick and want a little more vitamin C to fight off whatever's bringing you down. But when you do that, are you also appreciating the three grams of fiber and half a cup of water inside it? Probably not, but now that I told you an average orange contains all that stuff in addition to vitamin C, don't you feel even prouder for eating it?

See where I'm going with this? Healthy foods aren't just a one-trick pony. For example, many people turn to apples when they want more fiber in their diet, but apples also lower cholesterol and are loaded with both flavonoids and the phytochemical quercetin (both of which help attack DNA-damaging free radicals within your body that can be linked to cancer and other cell-damage issues). Or I've seen people snack on cherry tomatoes because they're low in calories, but they're also rich in folate, vitamin B6 and lycopene, an antioxidant that destroys free radicals and lowers your risk of stroke.

When you spend a second to really learn about and appreciate all the benefits you're getting from whatever healthy food you're eating, it raises the importance of that food in your mind. It makes it more valuable in your eyes because you recognize everything that it's bringing to the table for you.

But hey, I'm not expecting you to appreciate every single vitamin, mineral, and antioxidant in every single food you eat. I'm just asking you to appreciate the more obvious ones first, then get curious about what else is hiding inside your food that's secretly helping your health along the way. The more positive benefits you can associate with smart choices, the more likely you'll reach for them over less healthy foods later.

Appreciate every bite and sip—not just the first. Trust me, I'm sometimes guilty of eating way too fast, especially if I'm on the court or on the go and just need to fuel up. But when you slow things down enough to really chew your food and appreciate every bite, a few positive things happen along the way.

The most obvious is that you'll eat less without trying to. It takes roughly twenty minutes for your stomach to let your brain know it's full, so the longer you appreciate your food, the fewer bites and sips you'll sneak in between before your brain finally realizes your body has everything it needs nutritionally.

But I've found there's a side benefit to slowing it down when throwing it down, and that's this: if you take more time to chew your food (imagine a minimum of thirty times before swallowing, but don't feel the need to count if that's too much pressure—you can ballpark it!), you'll get a better sense of what's truly in the food you're eating.

What do I mean by that? Processed foods (like white bread, crackers, pretzels, hot dogs, and so on) have little to no nutritional value and typically break down in your mouth after just a few bites. That's because, to make these types of foods last longer on store shelves, they're stripped of a lot of fiber, vitamins, and minerals. However, more wholesome foods like raw fruits and vegetables, for example, usually take a little bit longer to chew because they're packed with more nutrients. The more often you practice appreciating every bite, the more likely you'll make the connection between which foods take a little extra time to chew because they're worth it—and which ones are not worth your time at all.

Appreciate the process you picked. Hey, I'm not a nutritionist, but I understand that there are better or worse ways to cook the same foods, and, let's face it, so do you. If I asked you what was healthier for you—steamed fish or fried fish—would you honestly not know? Of course you would, because everyone gets that when you pick a better way to prepare food over a less healthy way, you can strip away unhealthy fat and excess calories without changing the ingredients of the meal.

That's why, with each meal or snack, I want you to ask yourself (when applicable) if there was a better way it could've been cooked or prepared—and did you decide to go with the smartest, healthiest way? Not sure? Here's a quick cheat sheet from best to worst: steamed, broiled, baked, stir-fried, sautéed, fried, and deep fried.

If you picked the best possible choice, then give yourself credit and appreciate that you did. And if you didn't, that's okay too. I want you to appreciate the fact that you recognize that food could have been prepared better. Because when you acknowledge that, believe me, you'll be more likely to make a better decision the next time.

Appreciate—Your Activities

Most people complain when a muscle aches or they feel tired after exercise. When I'm sore or spent from playing tennis, working out, or doing some sort of physical activity, I may not always enjoy that feeling afterward, but it also reminds me that I feel that way because I was doing what's best for my body. I appreciate when I feel temporarily uncomfortable—because it reminds me *why* I feel that way in the first place.

It's really about how you look at it—this kind of attitude shift totally changes the game. From this point forward, I want you to appreciate how you feel after physical activity because it means you accomplished something. You threw something at yourself that's going to make you a little bit healthier the next day. It's proof that you put time into yourself because you deserve it.

But that feeling isn't the only thing I want you to consider appreciating when it comes to your activities. There are other things to be grateful for that can raise your confidence and remind you what you're capable of.

Appreciate what you have access to. It doesn't take much to burn fat, build lean muscle, and keep your heart healthy, and in the next section, I'll show you just how easy it is to do that with very little equipment. But that doesn't mean I don't want you to never consider other exercise options.

Maybe you live close to a park that has the most amazing trails to run on, or the building you live in has a gym. Maybe your job offers a gym membership, or you're lucky enough to live in a warmer climate that lets you be active outside more often. Or you live in a city where you get to walk every day, or your building has a challenging twelve-floor staircase you could climb. We all have access to something we could be appreciating, but the key is recognizing and taking advantage of those things, because when we seize the opportunities given to us, then even more come our way.

Appreciate what your body is made for. I may be fit for tennis and a few other sports, but that doesn't mean my body is perfectly in shape for every type of sport or activity—and neither is yours. Have a body that's built for running long distances but sinks like a stone when you try to swim? Too short for a certain sport but just the right size for another? Are you too top-heavy to jog, but have a broad upper body perfect for rowing? Not flexible enough (yet!) for yoga but have a pair of powerful legs for cycling?

That's what's beautiful about the human body—we're all built differently! And what might not make you the best at one activity might give you an edge with another. Instead of focusing on what activities you can't do as well because of your size, weight, height, or whatever, love what makes your body different and appreciate how that uniqueness may give you an advantage in certain activities.

Appreciate that you can participate. We've all heard the expression that we don't realize what we have until it's gone. That same logic applies to what you can do physically. Imagine for a second that you physically couldn't run anymore. That your muscles were too weak to lift an empty glass, let alone a dumbbell. That your lower back was so tight, you couldn't touch your knees if you bent over—forget about your toes!

The next time you're at a gym, a park, or any place where people are being active, take a second and just look around. Don't focus on anyone who might be in better shape than you. Instead, look for those who seem to be struggling with what you can do. Really let it sink in that you're blessed to be able to be active and exercise in the first place. Recognizing how lucky you are can put your mindset in a more positive place that helps you get more from whatever activity you choose.

Appreciate the results that aren't instantaneous. Getting in the best shape of your life through regular exercise and activity doesn't just happen overnight, and I know it sounds crazy to say this, but you should be thrilled about that.

Why would I say this? Well, think about it. Any achievement worth accomplishing typically takes plenty of effort and time. But whenever something is just handed to you—or you achieve it by taking the easy road—you really don't appreciate that achievement as much, do you? I mean, if you got an A+ on a math test but used a calculator to get all the answers, would you be *that* proud of yourself? What would you appreciate more—something that was just given to you for no reason, or something that you saved up and worked hard for?

Transforming your health and your physique by being more active may be a slow process, but it's one that is guaranteed to work if you're patient and persistent. Sure, you may not notice the results immediately, but before you know it, you'll be saying to yourself, "Oh my gosh, I'm getting stronger," or, "My legs look better in these shorts." It definitely doesn't happen overnight, but it will happen, and when it does, appreciating that it's meant to take time will give you a stronger sense of pride when it finally does.

Appreciate the time you have. I haven't met a single person who didn't tell me they were always super busy and barely had enough time in the day to get everything done. That's life, right? But the reality is you can always find time to improve yourself—it's all about wanting to do it.

Only *you* know how busy you really are, how much free time you *really* have, and what you're spending (or wasting) all those minutes on. Hey, no judgment here. All I'm asking you to do is appreciate the fact that you do have more time than you're probably giving yourself credit for. Appreciate the fact that you do have the amount of time that it takes to exercise because by acknowledging it (even if it's just to yourself), you'll be less likely to make excuses later that you don't have a minute to devote to staying fit.

However, I want you to also remember that there will be days that you have less time to give, so don't get down on yourself if you aren't able to devote the same amount of time to your goals every day—it all still counts. It's no different from when you put money into a savings account. What you put in may not always be the same amount, but it still adds up and compounds over time. Just appreciate the time you have to improve yourself, no matter how little or how much.

Appreciate that you tried. For me, there are days when I don't even want to move. When I'm so tired that the thought of playing tennis or doing anything active is out of the question. But even on the worst of days, if I get off my butt and force myself to try, the same thing always happens. After a few minutes, it starts to feel good. *I* start to feel good, and before I know it, I'll have pulled off a full workout or practice that I swore I didn't have the energy to do. Sure, maybe that day my performance was off, or I wasn't as quick or as energetic as I could have been—but I showed up. It's all about taking that first step and trying, even on the days you don't want to.

Let's own this right now. Are there going to be days when what you bring to your activities is subpar at best? Will there be moments when you cut a workout short because you have another priority that day? No doubt—and that's all good—but remember this.

Even during those days when you fall short of your expectations, appreciate yourself for showing up and not being marked absent. Appreciate that anything always beats nothing, and how on those days—so long as you're being honest about only having so much time to spend or energy to give—every little bit counts.

Appreciate—Who and What's Around You

Once I found out I had an autoimmune disease, it made me appreciate things I hadn't appreciated before. I found myself stepping back from what I was going through, and instead, I started to look at the other areas of my life and how blessed I was—particularly when it came to the people around me.

If you've already *observed* those around you, then you're already a little more aware about how blessed you are when it comes to who supports you and has your back through thick and thin. But just because those people are there now doesn't mean they'll always be there.

Every relationship takes work, whether it's for someone you've known forever or someone you've just met, but just because it's work doesn't mean it has to be overwhelming. Sometimes, all you really have to do to keep those relationships growing is spend a little time appreciating the people who are a part of your life in whatever way works for you.

Appreciate by actively listening. I don't care who you talk to, where they're from, or what they do. I believe everybody has something to teach us. But appreciating all that knowledge that's walking around you can't happen unless you spend more time using your ears than your mouth.

When you really think about it, most conversations play out like a tennis match, with words being hit back and forth. But most of the time, people aren't truly listening to the point the other person is trying to get across as much as they're just eagerly waiting for their turn to talk about themselves.

Instead of simply listening for your chance, take the time to appreciate the conversation—no matter who you're talking to—and really listen to what they have to say. In fact, challenge yourself not to spin the conversation back to you and to instead listen with intent—the intent being to ask a question that builds upon what that person was just telling you.

I know this one sounds easy at first, especially because you might think you already do this. But it's not until you make a conscious effort to actively listen that you suddenly realize most of your conversations have probably been tennis matches too. Just try spending the day approaching every conversation you have—

with anyone you meet—with the goal of trying to figure out what that person has to teach you. I guarantee you they'll walk away appreciating you more for really listening to them—and you might walk away appreciating what they shared.

Appreciate a moment—then remind those that made it a moment. I recently took up the hobby of going to escape rooms. I know, it's very nerdy. I absolutely love them because they let me compete with myself. They also remind me how we all have different ways of thinking through problems, because once you go in, most times to solve the puzzle, you have to think in an entirely different way than you might be used to in order to get out.

I do them a lot now with friends and family (my niece, brother-in-law, sister, and mom) and afterward, we'll take pictures, go out for dinner, and relive the whole thing over again. I even have a picture of my family looking scared running from a Tyrannosaurus rex (shot on a green screen), with Serena looking terrified but taking a selfie at the same time! These escape rooms have become a new way to create and share amazing and fun moments with the people I care about the most—and I think about them at different points of my week.

When was the last time a great memory popped into your head, or you saw or heard something—a picture, a song, something you found in your junk drawer—and it reminded you of a fun time you spent with someone. It doesn't have to be an amazing moment, just anything that just made you feel good or smile.

Instead of just enjoying that moment silently in your head and then letting it quickly pass, I want you to stop everything you're doing and give that memory your undivided attention so it lingers a little longer and doesn't just go in and out of your head. And then, reach out and remind whoever was attached to that moment.

You don't have to make much of an effort. A text, an email, a quick call—whatever's convenient at the time—but do it when you're reminded of that moment, if possible. It's all about sharing the moment with the actual person who made it a moment.

When you do this, you'll be floored by how it takes a positive memory and amplifies it, especially if that friend responds and starts remembering other details that you might've forgotten. But what's coolest of all is that it opens the door with that person to do something like that for you in the near future.

Appreciate those who got you here. Wherever you are right now, you didn't get there alone. I know I didn't, and when I consider everybody who's played a part in the life I've been blessed to have, it's overwhelming. Because when you really sit down with your thoughts to consider who made a difference in making your world better, I'm telling you, that list can start to add up fast.

Everybody has someone from their past who's had a positive influence on them. Maybe it was a teacher, an old friend, a neighbor, a past co-worker, or even just a person you met in passing a long time ago who happened to say or do something that somehow shifted you in a different trajectory.

Take a few minutes to make your list, and, if it's possible, reach out and thank that person who helped you move a little bit closer toward the goals you had for yourself. And if it's not possible, then just spend a moment acknowledging what they did—whether they realized it or not—and remind yourself how it sometimes takes just the smallest of actions to make the greatest impacts.

Appreciate by recognizing your rivals. Look, not everybody in life can be your friend. You don't have to be an athlete to be in competition with somebody, whether you want to admit you're competing with them or not. Maybe it's that person at work who's as eager as you are to impress the boss. Or that person at your gym who always seems to last a little longer on the treadmill than you. I could come up with other scenarios, but I think if you sit with the idea a bit, you could probably think of at least one person who you may have a little bit of a rivalry with, whether they know it or not.

If you don't, then congratulations on being a saint. But if you do, a little rivalry can be healthy when you're not obsessive about it. Sometimes we push ourselves a little harder when we're not in first place, and when we chase that faster horse, so to speak, it can make us run a little faster than we otherwise might have. We end up striving above and beyond what we thought we were capable of simply because we don't want the other person to win.

Keeping all that in mind, I want you to think about who your rival might be. But instead of letting jealousy turn your thoughts negative, appreciate the fact that someone exists who probably is fueling you to go further, then ask yourself what they may be doing that's allowing them to succeed in areas where you may not be doing so great. Better still, don't be afraid to ask them for help, especially if they're not really an enemy and are somebody who's achieved something you hope you can achieve one day.

Appreciate—Yourself

When I say this might be the hardest portion of the book, it's easy to see where I'm coming from, right? I mean, who can really do that? Who do you know who honestly appreciates themselves for who they are, both the good and the bad, warts and all?

Often, we're our own worst critic. Even if everybody else around is telling us what a great job we're doing or how proud they are of us, it's not easy to allow ourselves to believe and absorb all the hype. Maybe it's because we think it leaves us looking egotistical to accept all that praise, almost as if buying into it makes it sound like we're agreeing with them, almost as if we're saying, "Yeah that's right—I'm as good as you say I am."

If you don't appreciate yourself in some way every day, you can't move forward, no matter how much outside support you may have. You become your own anchor pulling yourself down instead of lifting yourself up. But I've always believed that our attitude toward life gets us to where we are—or aren't. So, if your attitude with yourself isn't the best, then you're keeping yourself from being your best, plain and simple.

Appreciate what makes you different. Why is it so easy to point out our flaws and so difficult to shine a spotlight on our strengths? I mean, if I asked you to write down five things that you wish you could change about yourself, then told you to jot down five things you love about yourself, which list would you write faster? That's what I thought—and that's not where I need your headspace to be.

Many times, most of the things we think are flaws or weaknesses are simply the things that make us unique—they make us who we are—but we might consider them shortfalls because we're comparing ourselves to everyone else. But that's not being fair to yourself. I do know this: there's not a single person out there who doesn't believe they have flaws, including the ones you think are flawless.

I dare you to find anybody who's 100 percent satisfied with everything that makes them different. Go ahead and take your time—I'll wait right here. You won't find that person because they don't exist, but that doesn't mean you should ever regard what makes you *you* as an imperfection. Instead, try to:

Embrace what you can't change—and own it. Look, there are certain things we may not like about ourselves that we can't fix—wanting to be taller or having huge feet, for example—but instead of obsessing over what you can't do anything about, appreciate how those things set you apart from everybody else and move on.

Acknowledge what you can change and do something about it—within reason. If some of the issues you have with yourself are things you can fix, then appreciate the fact that what you're not happy with *is* within your control to do something about. Give yourself a time limit to make progress, and if you miss that goal, then no problem. Instead of beating yourself up about it, reevaluate the situation, then set a new timeline—as long as you're making some sort of progress, it's all good. But if you do take that route, just remind yourself along the way that what you may not like also makes you one of a kind in the meantime.

Appreciate how healthy you already are. Being out of shape is one thing, but being in such poor health that you couldn't get into shape, even if you had the time to do it, well, that's an entirely different story altogether

Maybe you're not happy with where you presently are at physically, but your body probably has a lot more going for it than you're giving it credit for. And even if you're in the worst shape of your life, you need to keep in mind that you have something that someone who's not in the best of health wishes they had.

To really appreciate how healthy you already are, you need to take inventory of where you are health-wise. Run the numbers and checks on everything—your glucose levels, your cholesterol levels, your blood pressure, your eyesight, your hearing, how clear your skin is, how nice your hair is—it doesn't matter what you decide to appreciate so long as it's tied to your overall health. And if you're not sure, get a full physical and have your doctor point out what you're doing right versus doing wrong.

I didn't really appreciate what it was like not to have Sjögren's—until I suddenly had to live with it. So, give yourself moments to recognize the high points of your health.

Appreciate every loss. Sometimes, you need to learn a lesson, and you might not even know what that lesson is—until you fail.

I'll give you an example: I once played in an Olympic tournament and had lost first-round singles *and* first-round doubles. Up until then, I had never lost an Olympic doubles match, but everything that could possibly go wrong had. Yet despite those two tough losses, I was selected for mixed doubles. I was excited and so grateful that they believed in me, and I looked at the opportunity like a moment of redemption for me.

So, I got out there and played my best, even though my arm was a bloody pulp from my previous matches, but I finally started playing well. On paper, I was the stronger player and more experienced in the pairing, and we made it all the way to the finals. At the start, we were up 6–0, but sometime after that, mistakes were made and once they started, we just couldn't stop the bleeding. I had put a **lot** of effort into getting to this final and it wasn't easy. We ended up losing.

When that happened . . . boy, did I take it hard! I was like, "I did all this work, and for what? I mean, how much **more** work do I have to do?"

For years I complained about it because all I could think about was how it would've been my fifth gold medal. And am I still mad because I lost? Absolutely—I'm only human. But over time, I was finally able to appreciate the lesson within that loss. How I had been so focused on my partner making mistakes that I let it affect how I was playing—and it caused me to miss the final shot of the match. I realized, "Wow, no matter how crazy that day was, in the end, it had nothing to do with me not working hard enough until that point. It wasn't my commitment that caused me to lose—I simply missed the last shot of the match. In the end, all I can really do is be responsible for winning on *my* side of the court."

It was a simple lesson: it wasn't that I could've tried any harder prior to the match, but that it just came down to one single point that could've gone either way—but it was my lesson to learn, and I felt so much better afterward. The problem was it took me years to learn that lesson, and I wasted time and energy focusing on the failure instead of what I could've learned from it. That's why now, anytime I lose in any aspect of my life, instead of letting it **get me** down, I **break it** down instead to see if there's anything at all that I can learn from that loss.

Appreciating your failures isn't about making yourself feel bad by picking apart how or why you lost. That's not what I want you to do. It's about remembering that everything—including that loss—is just a moment. It's understanding that "Hey, I didn't ruin everything by making a mistake or failing, and that doesn't mean I should never try whatever it was I failed at ever again." It's about recognizing that you're not always winning in life—*nobody* is. It's about asking yourself questions: Were there any roadblocks that you could avoid next time? Were there mistakes that you could prevent when you try again? It's taking a few minutes to appreciate that loss and how it might help you pinpoint certain improvable aspects of yourself so that you approach that goal smarter the next time.

Appreciate when it's time to quit. Most of us go through life with the old adage drilled into our heads to never give up because quitters never win, and winners never quit. I'll admit that mantra has some merit! I don't want you to quit on yourself, or anything you feel passionate about that would enrich your life. But what I'm talking about is appreciating when it's time to quit certain things that just aren't working as well for you as they should be.

For example, when it comes to your diet, you could strive to eat the top-ten healthiest vegetables for your body on a weekly basis, but if broccoli and brussels sprouts are on that list and you hate both, then you may be just setting yourself up for failure. Skipping rope is an incredible way to burn calories, but if you lack the coordination and patience to twirl that rope, then you're going to spend more time tangled up in it than using it to burn a single calorie.

My point is this: you're going to see many suggestions of things to try in this book, as well as be encouraged to strive and explore other options that I haven't presented. But lean into what you like, whether that's certain nutritious foods, activities you like more than others, or healthy habits that excite you rather than make you struggle, and you'll be more likely to incorporate these smarter choices into your life.

In other words, don't worry about what you can't do, and appreciate what you can do—for now. Because trust me, once you begin seeing progress in yourself by leaning on the changes you can make, you'll eventually find the strength and curiosity to take on what may currently be a struggle for you later down the road.

CHAPTER 5

BALANCE

How many times have you heard someone say how important it is to find balance in your life? They're not wrong, but you have to watch how you take that advice. A lot of people struggle with creating a more balanced life for themselves, but if they ever feel they're not pulling it off as planned, they easily become frustrated.

Some think I'm an "overachiever," when all I really am is a woman who has many plates spinning at the same time. But show me a woman who doesn't, am I right? We all have our own plates to spin. And sure, mine might be different from yours, but what matters is that you can easily keep the plates that matter most—the ones that make the most significant impact on your life in terms of health, wellness, and happiness—effortlessly and always up in the air.

Sounds impossible? Sure it does, but that's probably because you think you must spin *all* of the plates that matter most to you *all* at the same time—and *all* of the time. Please! No one does that, and if they say they do, they're either just pretending they have it all together or are seriously stressed out and failing in other aspects of their life from trying to juggle too much. I learned a long time ago that trying to live by absolutes can sometimes be the fastest way to failure.

That's why my outlook on balance is a little unconventional. I don't believe it's possible to live a balanced life—because your life is *always* going to be unbalanced. Especially if you're striving to achieve something, trying new things, furthering your learning, having a family, etc. These types of situations (and many others) naturally create imbalance. Not always in a bad way, but they take up time, effort, and energy, which leaves you with less of all those things for other sometimes important endeavors.

Nothing has ever been "completely balanced" in my world—I mean, ever. Instead, all I ever try to do is create these little *moments* of balance for myself within the imbalance. What do I mean by that? Well, it could mean anything from being able to create a more balanced workout or to modify my diet on the fly—not perfectly, but just enough to matter—to understanding how to get a better night's sleep on the road or just finding the strength to ask for help when I need a lift in spirit. By coming to grips with the fact that my life is unbalanced, and how that's just how it is and always will be, I feel less stressed out in moments when things are far from perfect. I also know that feeling unbalanced simply means that change may be necessary in certain areas of my life, and that I should reprioritize those when it comes to what's vital—and which "plates" matter most. Plus, it enables me to adapt to any possible situation that may disrupt my healthy lifestyle because I know I'm going to fall short occasionally—and that's all good. That way, when I mess up by making the wrong choice, I don't dwell on it too much because I know I can always get it right the next time—or balance something else that day instead.

Now it's your turn to follow my lead. In this section, I'm going to ask you to consider making a variety of thoughtful choices with regards to your diet, exercise, and other aspects of your wellbeing. Do I expect you to pull all of them off? No. Just go in with the mindset that each one of these is nothing more than a "moment of balance." Techniques that you can try most of the time but that

I want you to fully expect to fail at certain points. Each is merely meant to help bring a little bit more balance into your life in a way that's more manageable and less stressful. The more you practice them, the closer you'll meet and exceed your lifestyle goals.

Balance—The Right Way

No one divides their day up and spends every minute doing things that are healthy twenty-four seven—and I mean no one. So, before you consider any of the options in this portion of the book, I need you to keep these three things in mind:

Just because you balanced it today—doesn't mean you have to balance it tomorrow. What I mean is you're going to pick something from this chapter to bring balance to, but when you succeed, don't feel pressure to keep it in balance from that point forward as you explore other ways to bring more balance to your life. I mean, that would be great, but I'm expecting you to "try these life-balancing tactics on for size." Feel free to jump around and try whatever might be easier to pull off that day. Eventually, you're not even going to have to think about some of these techniques—they'll just become second nature as you get used to them over time.

If you can "only" balance one thing that day, target a bad habit. For me, that's going to bed late. I have FOMO and hate going to bed when I should because it's the only time of the day when it's quiet with no demands. I love that time so much that I don't want it to end, but when I do that, it makes me not want to get up the next day on time—so I wake up late, which causes my whole day to become very unbalanced.

Often, it's the unhealthy things in your life that steal the time we would've spent on healthier things. Meaning, the same amount of time you spend doing something negative is the same amount of time you could be using to do something positive. So, if you can't decide what to balance on any given day, make a choice that minimizes the bad stuff, which will make more room for your healthy choices to grow.

It's the quality—not the quantity—that counts. Although I encourage you to try bringing as many aspects of your life into balance as possible, the goal is to find moments of balance *without* stressing yourself out. Stress is its own issue that I'll get into within the "Soothe" chapter of this book. The long and short of it is, if you start to feel too much pressure or anxiety to keep as many things in balance as possible, the negative health issues that come with stress can oftentimes far outweigh whatever positive changes you're making. That said, don't focus on the number of things you're balancing, and remember, one is better than none for the day.

Balance—Your Diet

Okay, here's the part where you think I'm going to throw out some strict dietary guidelines that you could *maybe* pull off for a couple of weeks before a night out with your friends or some upcoming holiday causes you to toss it all out the window and feel like a failure afterward. Well, I hate to disappoint you, but that's not happening. That's not how I live and not what I would expect you to do.

First off, *STRIVE* isn't a diet book, although if you're hoping to drop a few unhealthy pounds and look a lot better, that's just one of the results waiting around the corner if you follow the nutritional advice. Second, balancing your diet doesn't mean I'm asking for an entire overhaul of everything you eat from the time you wake up until you go to sleep. Because for me, it's just about observing what I'm doing wrong, appreciating what I'm getting right, and then trying to shift the balance in my favor a little bit every day by eating better instead of worse.

I'm serious, because personally, I'm a junk eater. I love donuts and pie, but other times, I really want pancakes. Right now (as I'm sitting here thinking about it), I'm obsessed with eating Hostess Snoballs, but my go-to are SweeTARTS. They were my first favorite candy since I was a little kid, and in a perfect world—where cavities didn't exist and you could eat candy without elevating your sugar levels—I would eat rolls of them every day if given the opportunity.

I love junk food, but instead of denying or ignoring that about myself, I embrace it and accept it. I never think for one second that I could go cold turkey from eating junk food (even though it would technically be the healthiest choice to make) because that's just not realistic whatsoever. And even attempting to quit junk food altogether would only make me more miserable than happy, just as I'm sure walking away for good from your bad nutritional cravings would be for you.

Instead of trying to replace *all* of the bad stuff with good stuff, I'm more about using a smarter approach to fuel your body that lets you have fun with your nutrition (whenever possible) while still allowing yourself what I like to call "options for joy." By balancing certain crucial elements of your diet using easy-to-incorporate suggestions, you're put on a better path without having to worry about breaking down and calculating every single meal.

Balances will help boost your performance, leave you looking a lot leaner, and give your body more of what it truly needs. Here's my approach to balancing aspects of your diet:

Balance when you eat. Whenever you wait too long between meals—or even worse, blow off a meal—what that tells your body is this: I'm starving and need to get something immediately!

If there's no food around, then it starts breaking down whatever it can find for energy. And as much as you might wish it would go after your body fat (oh, if only it worked that way!), it typically breaks down what you never want to lose—your muscles. Worse still, taking too long between meals can also cause you to crave even larger portions of food later, in addition to scaring your body into storing a larger number of calories from whatever you eat during your next meal as fat—even if that meal was 100 percent fat-free.

That's why, before you change anything about what you eat, what might be the most important thing to balance about your diet is how often you eat. What I mean is getting your body on an eating schedule by having a decent breakfast, then continuing to eat something every two to three hours afterward. Depending on when you wake up, a typical schedule might look like this:

- Breakfast: 7:00 a.m.
- Snack: 10:00 a.m.
- Lunch: 12:30 p.m.
- Snack: 2:30 p.m.
- Dinner: 5:00 p.m.
- Snack: 7:30 p.m.

When you balance your eating habits by putting yourself on a more reliable eating schedule, you break up your daily calories into much smaller increments throughout the day in a way that curbs binges and keeps your body from feeling the need to store excess body fat as often. That's because your body learns that it can count on you to fuel it every few hours, making it less likely to freak out and make you crave more food than you really need to eat—or bad-for-you foods that you shouldn't be eating in the first place.

Even if weight loss isn't your concern, you're still doing your body good by balancing your schedule, which helps your body digest what you're eating more efficiently. Your body isn't designed to handle everything all at once. It takes time to break down, shuttle, and store whatever nutrients are in the foods you're eating. But when you stick with a schedule that has you eating smaller meals more frequently, it allows your digestive system to do that job more efficiently. The pluses: your body gets to absorb even more nutrients from your food, in addition to keeping your metabolism elevated more often throughout the day, because digesting food burns calories.

Now, do I expect you to eat exactly at those times I just listed? Please, it's not an exact science, and I wouldn't say watching the clock all day long is very enjoyable, would you? All I'm suggesting is that you keep when you're eating in mind and see how your body feels when it's in balance timewise between meals.

Balance what's on your plate. In a perfect world, every meal or snack should have all three of the following to balance it out:

1. Lean protein
2. Healthy fat
3. Complex carbohydrates

This combination works in your favor for several reasons: One, your body digests each at a different speed—carbs get broken down and absorbed the fastest, followed by protein, then finally fats, which take the longest. By eating all three at the same time, your body gets a constant flow of energy that keeps you more mentally aware all day long, minus the usual highs and lows most people typically experience throughout the day. That balanced stream of energy also prevents you from feeling as hungry in between meals and keeps your blood sugar levels nice and even.

Why is that last point so important? Well, when your meals or snacks are out of balance and contain mostly carbohydrates (particularly simple carbohydrates, like cookies, chips, white pasta, white rice, or foods made from white flour, for example), those carbohydrates are quickly digested into sugars and absorbed into your bloodstream. To handle all that sugar, your pancreas releases a larger amount of insulin, a hormone that can increase how much fat your body stores and lower how much fat it burns. The more even you can keep your blood sugar levels by balancing what's on your plate, the less insulin your body releases, so your body stores less of what you eat as extra body fat.

For now, which types of food you choose to be able to say, "Yeah, I've got all three on my plate!" is up to you. (Trust me, I'll show you how to ramp things up as we go along.) But a few obvious sources of each include:

- Lean protein: fish, chicken, turkey, low-fat meats, dairy products, or a combination of grains/legumes.
- Healthy fats: nuts, seeds, all-natural peanut butter, avocados, certain plant oils (including canola, olive, peanut, walnut, sesame, and sunflower oils), and cold-water fish. (The fish also counts as a protein, BTW.)
- Complex carbohydrates: vegetables, fruits, or grains (such as oats, brown rice, or quinoa).

All that said, do you have to be precise with all three categories? Am I expecting you to count calories and grams? Nope, not at all. What I consider "balancing your plate" is all about eating a normal serving of each category, while simultaneously staying aware of what's on your plate from a macronutrient standpoint (healthy fats, lean protein, and complex carbohydrates).

Here are just a few ways you could keep your plate balanced if you're looking for a little inspiration until you get the hang of it.

Balance Your Breakfast With . . .

- A tablespoon of almond butter spread on one to two slices of rye bread, and a glass of milk.
- One whole-wheat bagel with a slice of tomato and two to three ounces of smoked salmon.
- An omelet made from one whole egg, three egg whites, and a handful of baby spinach along with tangerine slices on the side.
- A serving of oatmeal with sliced strawberries and a splash of flaxseed oil mixed in, and six to eight ounces of low-fat milk.
- An omelet made from one whole egg, three egg whites, and a handful of diced vegetables, along with a serving of diced fruit.
- A yogurt with blackberries and a whole-grain bagel.
- A whole-grain waffle, a handful of raspberries, and six to eight ounces of skim milk.
- Six to eight ounces of nonfat yogurt with a few crushed walnuts and a handful of blueberries stirred in.

Balance Your Lunch With . . .

- A mixture of three to four ounces of chopped chicken breast and a cup of gluten-free pasta sprinkled with olive oil and a side of snow peas.
- Tuna salad (mix spring-water tuna, a quarter cup of nonfat mayo, and some fresh dill) on two pieces of sprouted whole-grain toast.
- A three-ounce hamburger (lean), with a slice of cheddar cheese wrapped in a whole-wheat pita with spinach, avocado, and tomato inside.
- A three- to four-ounce serving of turkey breast on pumpernickel bread topped with lettuce, tomato, onion, and sunflower seeds, along with a half cup of mixed berries.

Balance Your Dinner With . . .

- A three- to four-ounce serving of a bottom round roast, a cup of long-grain rice, and a cup of steamed broccoli drizzled in olive oil.

- A three-ounce serving of fatty fish (mackerel, salmon, or tuna, for example), one yam, and a cup of steamed green beans.
- A three- to four-ounce serving of pork tenderloin, one sweet potato, and a cup of mixed greens drizzled in olive oil.
- A three- to four-ounce serving of filet mignon with mixed greens sprinkled with sunflower seeds and a cup of steamed cauliflower.
- A three- to four-ounce serving of shrimp and a cup of grilled peppers, tomatoes, and mushrooms (as kebabs), a half cup of couscous with a half ounce of toasted sesame seeds mixed in, and a cup of mixed greens drizzled in olive oil.
- A three- to four-ounce serving of chicken (grilled), a half cup of quinoa, and one cup of steamed broccoli.
- A three- to four-ounce serving of top round steak, one slice of sourdough bread with a slice of avocado, and a cup of snow peas lightly covered in olive oil.

Balance Your Snacks With . . .

- One to two rolled slices of Swiss cheese, one to two rolled slices of roast beef drizzled in olive oil, and an ounce of pistachios.
- One whole-grain bagel with all-natural peanut butter and a half ounce of sunflower seeds.
- A cup of cottage cheese mixed with a cup of blueberries and a half ounce serving of chia seeds.
- A glass of skim milk and one pear (sliced) coated with a tablespoon of almond butter.

Balance your fluids. Staying hydrated is another one of the most important things you absolutely need to bring into better balance as quickly as possible, no matter what your goals might be for yourself.

Forget about the fact that drinking enough water during the day can help you feel more satiated, keeping your appetite in check so you're less likely to crave unhealthy foods or eat more calories than your body really needs during meals. For me, it's all about what that water is really doing behind the scenes.

Literally every system throughout your entire body needs water to operate properly. Water is working hard to help shuttle vitamins, minerals, and other nutrients to your cells. It's responsible for flushing out toxins, managing your blood pressure, and regulating your body temperature on top of cushioning your organs and joints against shock and injuries.

It's so crucial that letting yourself lose as little as one percent of your body weight in water can disrupt your body's metabolism (so you burn fewer calories all day long) and prevent you from delivering as much oxygen throughout your body (which can lead to fatigue that impacts your all-day activity). From an energy standpoint, that loss can lead to a 10 to 20 percent decrease in your performance according to most experts.

Personally, I like to start my morning with a sixteen-ounce glass of water, then I'll end the day with another sixteen ounces of warm water with lemon because I find it both tasty and comforting. I'll also have sixteen ounces directly after lunch and dinner (not during my meals—I do it afterward) and that takes me to sixty-four ounces. Anything I might drink on top of that is a bonus, but that's what helps me keep track without ever thinking about it. So, what's the best way for you to balance out your fluids?

- I could go old school and tell you to drink at least eight to ten eight-ounce glasses per day.
- I could tell you to weigh yourself every morning and have you drink half your body weight in ounces daily. Meaning, if you weigh 150 pounds, that would be 75 ounces (150 divided by 2 equals 75), for example.
- Or I could remove the math altogether and just insist that you always have a water bottle close by with at least sixteen ounces in it. That way, you can sip from it all day long from morning until night.

Honestly, any of these three scenarios would probably get you to drink more than you're presently doing, since most people typically walk around dehydrated and never even realize it. Whatever you pick will probably balance your fluid intake more than your current state, but I will offer a few suggestions, regardless of which path you choose:

Don't wait until you're thirsty to drink. By then, you're already dehydrated and your body's now busy doing your job for you, pulling water from wherever it can find it—your kidneys, your stomach, your colon, you name it. When you remember that every cell in your body has water in it, you can just imagine what price you're paying for all that borrowing your body is doing within itself. Trust me—it's not worth the price.

Don't wait until you start your day. Every morning, you're already behind the power curve because you're waking up dehydrated—and that's before you head to the bathroom. It's the reason I insist that before you reach for anything else—coffee, tea, juice—drink at least a full glass of water. In fact, put a glass by your bed that's ready to go in the morning so you have something to sip as you wake up and think about what you must get done that day.

Don't settle for the traditional eight to ten glasses. Will you somehow shift yourself out of balance if you drink too much as opposed to drinking too little? In my opinion, not at all—especially if you:

- **Love your coffee, or drink on occasion:** Caffeinated drinks and alcohol are diuretics, so when you drink them, they pull water from your body. It roughly takes about two cups of water to rehydrate from just one cup of coffee or an alcoholic drink, so have a glass of water handy when drinking either.

- *Exercise or play a sport:* If you're active on a regular basis (which if you're not, you will be once you get into the next section, "Balance—Your Activities"), the minimum amount you should shoot for is ten to twelve glasses daily. That's about ninety-six ounces a day. My best advice is to boost your numbers for better balance: You could drink an extra six to eight ounces about every fifteen minutes as you participate in a sport, work out, or engage in anything active (yard work, playing with your kids outside, etc.). Or weigh yourself right before your workout, then after you're done, weigh yourself again. Every pound you've lost is most likely from water loss, so drink a pint (sixteen ounces) of water per pound to bring your fluids back into balance.

- *Live or work where it's warm:* If you spend any time in a location that's hot (outside in the heat, or even just an over-heated building, for example), you could be losing up to two glasses worth of sweat an hour without even realizing it. If that's you, I recommend drinking at least four to six ounces of water before heading into the heat, then continuing to drink about six to eight ounces every ten to fifteen minutes to stay balanced.

Balance what's within your reach. We're all creatures of convenience, which means, if given the choice, we're reaching for whatever's closest to us instead of whatever might be a little more out of reach.

Hey, there's nothing wrong with that—the path of least resistance, right? But here's the thing: if you're smarter about what's around you foodwise—I don't mean just what you eat and drink but even what you use to eat and drink—you can sort of "rig the game" in your favor to make healthier choices without really having to think too much about it.

I'm not saying get rid of all your junk food, by the way. Remember my promise? Make it easy, enjoyable, and exciting? There's nothing enjoyable about getting rid of everything you love to eat. All I'm suggesting is to consider whether there's a way to bring a little more balance to your "access" of foods that aren't that great for you. That said, here are just a few ways to keep your nutrition on point by balancing aspects of your eating before you ever take a bite.

Bring balance to your food stashes. Typically, if you're going through your fridge or pantry, you're not doing it because you're curious about what's inside—you're heading in there because you're hungry. That means everything is up for grabs, and let's face it, we tend to make poorer choices because we're famished and looking to fill up quick. Changing the landscape a little bit can tip the odds in your favor by raising the chances of you eating smarter—if you take time to set the stage the right way.

Do a one-for-one switch out. We all have a ratio of good versus bad foods in our fridges and pantries. Try taking a quick tally to see what percentage of your food is healthy versus—let's face it—crap. It doesn't have to be perfect—just get an estimate (twenty-to-eighty, thirty-to-seventy, fifty-to-fifty, whatever it is). Then, every time you shop, change those numbers by looking in your grocery cart, checking the ratio, then tweaking it so it's a better good-to-bad ratio that you'll have at home. After just one or two trips, your ratio at home will swing in your favor. (Just be sure to take a new estimate every two weeks so that you're always rebalancing.)

Look for a "lesser of two evils" exchange. Look, the bad stuff is in there because you like it for a reason. If it's because you love something salty or sweet, consider other foods that may satisfy that craving. Like them because they're easy to throw in your bag on the go? Then find something that's equally convenient but less nutritionally disastrous. Is it prepackaged? Then see if there's a perishable version that's not heavily processed and packed with preservatives.

Try a "less is more" approach. Grab an unhealthy food from your fridge or pantry, write down its net weight in ounces, then challenge yourself to look for a smaller version of it in the store. I'm not gonna lie. Smaller versions of most products aren't always the best buys in terms of price, but then again, think about this: Would you rather save a buck by purchasing that two-pound bag of pretzel sticks? Or would you rather lose a buck buying a smaller size, but decrease your risk of eating a bigger portion, or more portions than you should? Trust me, less is more—meaning *more* beneficial to your overall health.

Finally, switch out your tableware. Can something as simple as reorganizing your dishes so that your bigger plates, bowls, and glasses aren't as easy to grab make that big of a difference? Absolutely, because when most people sit down to eat, they don't consider portion sizes as much as just filling up their plate.

By switching out larger tableware for smaller dishes, glasses, and containers, you'll unconsciously eat fewer calories than usual while still satisfying your appetite, even if you feel the need to finish your plate. By the way, when I say, "switch out," I literally mean putting your biggest tableware on the highest possible shelf of your kitchen cabinets so it takes a stepladder to reach them.

Balance—Your Activities

A lot of people think that in order to reshape your body—to achieve stronger muscles, a healthier heart, and way less excess body fat—it takes being active seven days a week or pushing yourself through seriously hard workouts every single time. But that's not the case at all.

What usually matters is making sure you're being a little more active than you are right now. Because if you're not satisfied where you're at physically, chances are you don't quite have the balance locked down on your activities just yet. But you will, I promise you.

First things first: visit a doctor for a health screening to make sure you're healthy enough to start a program. Once you get the green light, there are several areas of fitness to keep balanced if living a longer, healthier life—and looking good while you're living it—is your goal.

Balance your muscles. You absolutely need to be doing some form of resistance training, which is when you work a muscle (or group of muscles) against some form of resistance so that they break down from fatigue and stress, then rebuild themselves to be better than before (bigger, stronger, leaner, etc.). But what type of resistance training you choose is up to you.

Whether that resistance comes from performing exercises with machines, dumbbells, barbells, stretch cords, or just your own body weight—your body really doesn't care. So long as you're using some form of resistance that forces your muscles to contract (and fatigue) by making them repeat a movement a certain number of times, then you're all good.

What's the point? Especially if you don't have any interest in being stronger and fitter? I'll get into the details later as to why resistance training is critical to your health, but in a nutshell, the more lean muscle you have, the longer your metabolism stays elevated. That's because lean muscle uses energy in order to maintain itself (about three times more calories than body fat). That perk alone causes your body to burn more calories—and unwanted body fat—all day long, even when you're not exercising at all or even when you're asleep.

How many times a week? According to the American College of Sports Medicine, the best balance for the average adult is training each major muscle group two or three days a week, then resting them at least forty-eight to seventy-two hours in between so your muscles can heal. If you're working your muscles less or more than that, you're creating an imbalance that's preventing you from seeing results by either not training your muscles often enough, or by overworking them to the point where they never get a chance to rest and rebuild.

How many times should you do each exercise? Doing an exercise once is called a *repetition* (or *rep*). A group of consecutive reps performed without rest is called a *set*. But how many reps and sets you should do depends on your goals.

If you want noticeably stronger muscles, I recommend using a heavier weight (or resistance) that only lets you do between six to ten reps. If you want more muscular endurance, using a lighter weight that lets you do fifteen to twenty reps is better. Most experts prefer the middle ground to get the best of both worlds. That means using a weight that only lets you do eight to twelve reps before your muscles fatigue to the point that they can't do any more reps.

As for sets, it's tricky because the American College of Sports Medicine feels that doing any exercise for two to four sets is best, although the general consensus is that performing even just one set of an exercise can still be effective, especially for beginning or older exercisers.

So, what should *you* do? Well, despite what some fitness experts may tell you, there is no such thing as the one and only perfect workout. That's because the more you use the same routine over and over again, the faster your body adapts to it, to the point where it stops becoming stronger, fitter, and healthier. I'll give you a solution for that later, but for now, let me give you a place to start.

Honestly, I do try and love everything when it comes to resistance training, but my attitude has always been to utilize as many functional exercises as possible that not only build strength but challenge your core and balance at the same time. That's why the workout I'm recommending uses six multi-joint moves that keep your entire body constantly engaged.

But to make things interesting, you'll move from one exercise to the next with little to no rest in between. This not only helps you burn more calories *as you exercise* by keeping your heart rate elevated but also depletes your oxygen levels faster and more thoroughly. This forces your body to use even more oxygen than usual to bring itself back to a normal state after exercise (with some of those jobs being to bring your hormone and oxygen levels—as well as your body temperature and heart rate—all back to normal). Because your body burns about five calories in order to consume just one liter of oxygen, the more oxygen it needs to make things right again, the more calories you'll burn long after the workout's done and forgotten about.

If that sounds intense, know that this routine only takes twenty minutes a day, three times a week (resting forty-eight to seventy-two hours in between workouts). Could you do more than that? Sure, but I like to work smarter and not longer than I have to. That's why, for now, keeping it simple is the best way to bring your body back into balance.

Is this for beginner, intermediate, or advanced exercisers? All three, actually. The way it's designed, if any move is too difficult, you can choose to do a dialed-down version of it. And, if it feels too easy, just use the harder version that's a little more intense.

Do I need to warm up my muscles first? Yes. Doing any low-intensity activity for three to five minutes will help increase blood flow to your joints and muscles, making them more pliable and ready for what's ahead. If you don't have any equipment, you can walk in place and pump your arms back and forth, jog in place, or just pretend to skip rope. If you have a piece of stationary equipment (a treadmill, stationary bike, stair-climber, etc.), set it at a low speed or level and use it for three to five minutes.

Do I need any equipment? Just a pair of dumbbells. If you have a few different pairs, that's perfect. But if you don't, buy a set you can press over your head from a standing position about eight to twelve times. Grab a pair of dumbbells (one in each hand) and raise them up to the front of your shoulders (palms facing forward, elbows pointing down). Keeping your back straight, press the weights above you by straightening your arms, lower them back down to your shoulders and repeat.

The Circuit

This full-body circuit is composed of six exercises that, ideally, you'll do back-to-back with no rest in between. I want you to do eight to twelve repetitions per exercise. After you finish the circuit, you'll rest for sixty to ninety seconds, then repeat the whole six-move circuit once more—then you're done. You'll do this routine three times a week, resting a full day or two in between (so exercise on Monday, Wednesday, and Friday, for example.)

Now, depending on your skill and comfort level, you can tweak this circuit to work best for you.

For example:

If you need a break:

- Try resting a little longer between circuits (ninety to one hundred twenty seconds, or two to three minutes).
- Try resting between each exercise (up to thirty to sixty seconds).

If you want a challenge:

- Try resting a little less between circuits (thirty to sixty seconds, fifteen to thirty seconds, or don't rest at all).
- Try repeating the circuit three or four times instead of twice.

The Exercises

1. Dumbbell Squat

(Works the quadriceps, hamstrings, gluteus maximus, lower back, and calves.)

Stand straight with a dumbbell in each hand and your feet spaced hip-width apart, knees unlocked. Your arms should hang straight down from your sides, palms facing in.

The move: Slowly bend your knees and squat until your thighs are parallel to the floor. Push yourself back up into a standing position and repeat.

My advice: Try keeping your knees directly above your toes, but don't let them extend past your feet as you go. At the top of the movement, straighten your legs but don't lock your knees.

Need a break? Do a body-weight squat. Instead of holding a pair of dumbbells, just let your arms hang down by your sides or cross them in front of you.

Need a challenge? Spend three to four seconds to lower yourself down, then three to four seconds to raise yourself back up, and/or pause at the bottom of the exercise (when your butt is closest to the floor).

2. Burpee

(Works the quadriceps, hamstrings, gluteus maximus, core, shoulders, chest, triceps, and calves.)

Stand with your feet shoulder-width apart and arms down by your sides.

The move: Quickly squat down as deep as you can and place your hands on the floor shoulder-width apart. Keeping your hands on the floor, kick your legs out straight behind you—you should end up in the top portion of a pushup. Bend your elbows and do a quick push-up, then immediately pull your knees back in to your chest—so your feet end up between your hands. Then immediately jump as high as you can, extending your arms above you. That's one rep!

My advice: The exercise should just flow and be one continuous move-ment that's a combination of a squat, a push-up, and a standing jump.

Need a break? There are a few ways to dial down the intensity:

- Once you land, take a quick pause before repeating the exercise.
- Drop to your knees to do each push-up.
- Instead of kicking your legs back and jumping them forward, you can walk them into place.
- Don't jump at the end of the move and just stand up.

Need a challenge? There are also a few ways to bring even more to this powerful exercise:

- Each time you jump, tuck your knees up toward your chest.
- Pause for a second or two at the bottom of the push-up.
- Each time you jump, twist yourself in midair to either the left or right.

3. Dumbbell Deadlift

(Works the back, quadriceps, hamstrings, core, and calves.)

Stand straight—feet hip-width apart—with a pair of dumbbells on the floor along the outsides of your feet. Bend your knees and grab the dumbbells with a neutral grip (palms facing in).

The move: Keeping your head up and back flat, slowly stand up until your legs are straight, keeping the weights close to your legs as you go. Lower the weights back down to the start position.

My advice: Don't stare down at the weights or at your feet. Look forward instead for better balance.

Need a break? Instead of lowering the weights down to the start position, only bend down about halfway.

Need a challenge? Try a unilateral deadlift instead. To do this, place a single dumbbell along the outside of your left foot. Bend your knees and grab the dumbbell with your left hand (letting your right arm hang down at your side), then do the exercise as described for the required number of repetitions. Then switch positions and perform the exercise again (this time holding the dumbbell with your right hand).

4. Push-up

(Works the chest, shoulders, triceps, and core.)

Place your hands flat on the floor, shoulder-width apart, then straighten your legs behind you (keeping your weight on your toes). Your body should be a straight line from your head to your heels.

The move: Keeping your arms close to your sides, bend your elbows and lower yourself down until your upper arms are parallel to the floor, then immediately push yourself back up.

My advice: Don't look at your arms. Instead, stare straight down. Keeping your head in line with your back helps with balance and prevents you from accidentally straining your neck muscles.

Need a break? If regular push-ups are too difficult for now, you have a few options:

- Do the exercise with your knees on the ground.
- Lower yourself down as slowly as possible, but don't push yourself back up. (Just get back into the start position whatever way is easiest for you each time.)

Need a challenge? Put your feet up (on the bottom step of a staircase or a stable box) so that your head is lower than your feet in the push-up position.

5. Dumbbell Lunge

(Works the quadriceps, hamstrings, gluteus maximus, lower back, core, and calves.)

Stand holding a dumbbell in each hand, arms hanging straight at your sides, palms facing in.

The move: Keeping your back straight, take a big step backward with your left foot, and lower yourself down by bending your right knee until your right thigh is parallel to the floor. Push yourself back up into a standing position, then repeat the exercise by stepping back with your right leg. That's one rep!

My advice: Don't stare down at your feet (which can cause you to lose your balance). Instead, always look forward.

Need a break? Try doing the exercise without dumbbells, or instead of lowering yourself down the full amount, just go about half as far.

Need a challenge? Try pausing at the bottom of the move for two or three seconds, and/or keep the weights pressed over your head.

6. Dumbbell Row

(Works the back, biceps, and core.)

Stand with your feet shoulder-width apart, knees slightly bent, and a dumbbell in each hand. Keeping your back flat, bend forward at the waist until your torso is almost parallel to the floor, arms hanging down with your palms facing in toward each other.

The move: Without moving your torso, squeeze your shoulder blades together, then pull the dumbbells up to your sides. Slowly lower the dumbbells back down until your arms are straight once again. That's one rep.

My advice: Don't bend your neck to look up and forward. Instead, keep your neck in line with your back.

Need a break? Instead of holding your torso almost parallel, bend forward until your torso is about halfway from parallel, and/or only pull the dumbbells up halfway.

Need a challenge? Try raising one dumbbell at a time (which will challenge your balance) and/or pausing at the top of the exercise for three to four seconds.

Balance your cardio. In addition to doing some form of resistance training, the Centers for Disease Control and Prevention recommend that the average person do at least 150 minutes a week of cardiovascular activity at a moderate intensity. So, if balance is your goal, then what exactly does that mean?

Cardiovascular exercise (or *cardio*) is any activity that increases your heart rate. Not a runner? Aerobics classes really not your thing? That's fine because your body doesn't care how you make your heart work a little harder. What counts is participating in any activity that raises your pulse between 50 to 70 percent of your *maximum heart rate* (MHR) and keeps it there throughout the entire session.

How do you figure out what your MHR is? Easy. Just subtract your age from 220. For example, if you're 45, then your MHR would be 175 (220 minus 45 equals 175.)

Don't want to do the math? Then just use this trick: remember when I mentioned the Rate of Perceived Exertion Scale in the "Observe" chapter? If you feel you're pushing yourself between a five or six (where you can talk during the activity but singing would be too hard), then you're most likely between 50 to 70 percent of your MHR. Easy, right?

What cardio should *you* pick? There are hundreds of ways you could get a cardiovascular workout besides using gym equipment (treadmills, stair-climbers, rowers, stationary bikes, etc.) or the usual suspects, like jogging, swimming, and biking. On top of that, playing a sport obviously counts, as well as other pulse-raising activities like kayaking, ice-skating, and even dancing. And yes, keeping up and playing with your kids even works too.

To be fair, certain activities definitely blast more calories, such as skipping rope, swimming, stair sprinting, and running—but are any of those really your thing? Because if they're not, then you're more likely to quit doing them.

Sure, there are more popular versions of cardio out there to try, but if they're too difficult or too boring for you, it will only make it harder for you to hit that 150-minute requirement every week to stay balanced. That's why your best bet is sticking with whatever cardio options keep you curious and coming back for more.

To reach 150 minutes a week, most experts suggest breaking that number down into five 30-minute sessions to start. Those five sessions don't have to all be the same activity. In fact, I would prefer they weren't. Every cardiovascular activity works a different mix of muscle fibers and challenges your body in different ways. So, the more variety you can bring, the more balanced your body will be.

Balance your steps. Walking may rank as one of the lowest cardiovascular exercises out there in terms of burning calories—you're talking around one hundred calories per mile, which is about two thousand steps—but it's easy on the joints, it's the least risky in terms of injury, and you can do it all day long. For all those reasons, it pays to plod along every chance you can.

If you've observed your steps, you're already familiar with how many you typically take in a day. But to bring things into balance, it's time to step things up a bit—literally. They say the average person walks around five thousand steps a day, but who wants to be average? I know you don't. That's why I want you to raise your daily total to at least seven thousand five hundred or to as much as ten thousand a day.

Now, before you say that's impossible, remind yourself how often you either sit or stand during the day. Even the most inactive person is perfectly capable of pacing or walking in place instead, which, by the way, still counts! But if you want a few ideas on how to always hit that total, these clever tried-and-true tricks can help:

- Place things that you use multiple times a day at the farthest spot of your house possible (for example, your car keys, the remote, etc.). Then, after you use it once, put it right back.
- Make a point of always grabbing the farthest (but safest) parking space possible.
- Promise yourself you'll never talk on the phone unless you're walking at the same time.
- Show up for appointments fifteen minutes early, then use the time before your appointment to walk or pace.
- Instead of walking in the straightest path possible wherever you need to go, consider circling around it.
- When shopping, walk every single aisle—and not just the ones that have what you need. Then, when you come home, don't carry

as many bags as possible into the house but bring them in one at a time so you have to make more trips.

- Instead of sitting on the bleachers watching your kids play sports, walk up and down the sidelines as you watch.

Balance—Who and What's Around You

Who we surround ourselves with is a choice, and you want people who add value to your life.

I think we have people in our lives for different reasons and even for different seasons. But when you're talking about those who are there for most (or all) of our moments—the people we bring into our circle and keep there—those are the ones who must provide some value. Those are the relationships that need to be mutually beneficial for both of you, because if it's uneven—then call it whatever you like, but—it's not really a fair relationship, right?

Maintaining that balance isn't always easy, because sometimes it means having to walk away from people we might care for but who are potentially toxic for us and/or might not have our best interest at heart. To make matters worse, that person could be someone we can't just walk away from, such as family members, bosses and co-workers, teachers, or neighbors.

But you still have a choice. You still have a say when it comes to how much time you spend with them and the direction of the conversations. You have more power when it comes to tipping the scales than you might realize—it's just a question of being ready to strike a balance with those in your circle.

Balance by being true to your values. In the past, whenever I've found myself in a situation that was toxic, unhealthy, or just not ideal, it started with forgetting what I stood for. When you're not sure what your values are, you're inevitably going to have a lot of things in your life that you may not want, and that includes people who may not be the healthiest for you.

A good example of this is when you're dating someone you think is perfect, but then they start doing things that make you feel uncomfortable or unhappy, things that leave the relationship feeling out of alignment. When you're not firm on what you stand for, you might let those things slide, and soon, those things making you uncomfortable just become accepted behaviors. The problem with that is there's nothing harder to change in a relationship, because that person can always come back to you and say: "Well, if it was fine back then—why isn't it fine now?"

But when you stick to your guns about what your values are— what you like and what's acceptable to you—people like that never find their way into your life. And if they're already in your circle, staying true to yourself gives that person little choice but to either change or eliminate themselves from the relationship.

It's honestly one of the easiest and most kindhearted ways to remove people who aren't as healthy for you, especially if you're nonconfrontational. There doesn't have to be shouting or embarrassment. All it takes is telling people how you feel, and then asking them what they think—but stay firm. Just telling the truth about who you are and what you stand for starts to eliminate people in your life who shouldn't be there.

Balance by rationing your time. If you can't avoid everybody who's toxic in your life, you still have some control over how much time you give them. That's why I want you to consciously make an effort to spend more time with those who believe in you and less time with those who don't. But when I say, "more time" and "less time," what I really mean is this:

- When it comes to the good ones, "more time" means as much time as possible.
- When it comes to the bad ones, "less time" means I want you to literally ration out how many minutes you're going to give that negative person—and stick to it.

Before you start doing this, try keeping track each day of how many minutes you're devoting between people who are healthy for you versus unhealthy.

Those numbers tell a story—and that's your life story. They reveal how much time you're giving to people who aren't bringing anything positive to your table. People who may only show up in your life when they want something or need to complain instead of support you.

Once you see how you spend your time, change the numbers in your favor by only giving the toxic less than five minutes once a day at the very most—then start dialing that number back even further. Eventually, the less time you give a toxic person, the more likely they are to move on to someone else who has more time to listen to their woes or give them what they want.

Balance by opening up to your unhealthy friends. Throughout this book, you're going to begin changing aspects of your life, but some of what you hope to accomplish probably *won't* be what some of your friends are doing for themselves.

Why is that? Because we all have those few individuals in our lives whom we adore—those who support us and would do anything for us—BUT . . . they don't exactly practice what we're hoping to preach. I'm talking about friends who haven't eaten anything green since the last time something spoiled in their fridge, or the ones who think walking to the bathroom to pee between binge-watching Netflix counts as exercise. You love them, and they're not ever leaving your inner circle. But honestly, they're tough to be around when you're trying to pull off a healthier lifestyle.

The truth is, you *are* who you hang out with, but that doesn't mean you have to follow the herd mentality. And hey, I get it. It's hard to stick with healthy habits around certain friends without feeling like you're coming off preachy and superior. But recognize that the *only* way you'll feel like *that* person is if you *act* like that person.

That said, if certain friends aren't making healthy choices around you, then you just do what you need to do for yourself. If that's avoiding certain situations (like going out to eat, or partying all night when you want to exercise the next morning), so be it. All I ask is that you try a little honesty with them first. If they truly have your back, then telling them why certain situations may be more challenging for you shouldn't be a problem they can't work around. And if they don't understand your goals for yourself, re-member that what you're ultimately trying to do is live a happier and healthier life. Any friend who wouldn't support that wish may not really be your friend after all.

Balance—Yourself

Time is important and one of the few things in life we can't get back after we spend it. As for how you spend it? Well, that's entirely up to you. But it's important to remember that what's bad for you *and* what's good for you both fight for your hours, minutes, and seconds. But it's *you* who decides who gets them.

There's something I always tell myself when I'm on the court: "In the time I'm spending *missing* this ball, I could be spending the same amount of time *making* this ball." And that mantra pretty much applies for everything in your life.

The same afternoon you lie on the couch wishing your body

looked better is the same afternoon you could've put toward going to the gym and making it look better. The same lunch hour you blew eating unhealthy foods is the same lunch hour you could have used eating healthier foods. Whatever time you spend dwelling on a negative thought could be spent basking in a positive one.

Could you ever replace everything that's bad for you with what's good for you? Absolutely not, and the pressure of trying to pull that off, day after day after day, only causes unnecessary stress and anxiety that you don't need. Just remember that no matter which steps you try in this entire section (and throughout this book), they will help you achieve more moments of balance in your life than were there before.

Balance by taking away two plates. There's a certain pride that comes with handling more than the average person, isn't there? Is that you? The type who knowingly and willingly bites off more than they can chew, just so they can keep busy.

Sure, it's sometimes satisfying to spin a lot of plates, whether it's to brag about how we're superwoman, or just to feel productive knowing we're getting so much done. Sometimes we have no choice because so many other people may count on us. But each of those plates comes with a price, and that's a certain amount of stress.

I'm with you though. I sometimes forget how many plates I'm whirring until, eventually, one either crashes to the floor or I wear myself out to the point of exhaustion. Sometimes I feel I need to keep them all going because I don't want to let anyone down. I have to remind myself that my "fear" of disappointing others will eventually lead to disappointing myself if I've overwhelmed myself to the point where it's impossible to do it all.

Recently, I told Serena that every time I reply to one email, ten more always come back in. That whenever I've tried to clear up my schedule over the last few years, it always seems to go awry again. But deep down, I also know why it keeps happening. Being overcome by life is inevitable when you don't consciously choose your priorities wisely. You really have to choose what's honestly top priority and what matters to you.

That's why I want you to count all your plates, then find two—not one, but two—that you can either step away from or pass on to someone else. If you're not sure which two, then ask yourself:

- **Do I have to spin this plate all alone?** Meaning could you ask someone to help you split the time spinning it?
- **Could I delegate this plate to someone else?** Sometimes pride keeps us from admitting that someone else could probably do the job too—maybe even better.
- **Do I really need to keep this plate spinning—or will it probably spin all by itself?** There's usually at least one plate we keep spinning that we could've stopped spinning long ago.

Balance by adding two plates. Conversely, there are also some people who are fully able to take on more within their own lives. But their fear of failing, lack of organization or interest, or worries about the stress that comes with those extra roles prevent them from even considering it.

A big part of balance is feeling fulfilled and living up to one's potential, which is why it's important to be honest with yourself about whether you're doing as much as you could to move yourself forward in life. Unhappiness can easily come from being unbalanced in a way that causes you to underachieve and not realize your dreams. The very act of just going for it—even if the extra plates you're adding into your life come crashing down occasionally—can still give you a certain satisfaction in failing when you know you're at least trying.

So, if you feel as if you could be doing more, then find two plates you could add into your day (or week) by asking yourself:

- **Is there anything I've been avoiding intentionally?** It doesn't matter what it is or why you've waited so long to tackle it. What's important is that most things we put off are things we're afraid of or think we'll never get a handle on. Seeking out these types of plates to spin not only lets you finally check them off your to-do list but also lets you build your self-esteem and makes you more likely to tackle even more tasks with confidence.
- **Could someone else benefit from this as well?** There are always plenty of tasks that can also balance the life of someone else, such as that of your spouse or partner, someone you work with, a friend, a neighbor, etc. Try to choose plates that could directly or indirectly affect someone you care about in a positive way once you've gotten them spinning.

Balance by getting enough z's. So how much sleep is considered "enough"? I know there are days when I feel fine with less than eight hours and others where I'm so wrecked, I would sleep the day away if I could. But according to many sleep experts, most people need around seven to nine hours of quality sleep a night. But do they get it? That's tricky, especially because there's research out there that the average person overestimates how much shut-eye they get by about forty-eight minutes.[1]

The easiest way to decide if you're sleeping enough is to gauge how well you function during the day. Finding it tough to remember things or focus? Yawning often? People calling you out on often being edgy or grumpy? Can't stay alert during moments that you should? If that's you, then you're probably robbing yourself of quality sleep somewhere, but there are a few tricks you can try:

- Try going to sleep and waking up at the same time each day (even on the weekends or days off) since sleeping in—even just for a day—can often interfere with your sleep cycle for the whole week.
- Try adjusting where you sleep so that it's not too cold or too warm. Think "cool" instead (between sixty to sixty-eight degrees if possible), which helps most people nod off faster and promotes a deeper sleep. If you can't mess with the thermostat for some reason, you can still cool yourself down by putting a small pillow in your freezer a few hours before bedtime, then tucking it between your knees.
- Step back from anything stimulating at least one hour before you go to bed—that includes a difficult book, work, your phone, tablet, or TV (or any electronic device, since light stimulates your eye's photoreceptors and can signal your brain to stay awake).
- If you have trouble falling asleep after twenty to thirty minutes, just get up instead of being upset with yourself, but leave your lights either low or off. Then pick something peaceful to do until you start feeling tired, like stretching, listening to relaxing music, or reading something light.
- Finally, don't use your bed for anything but sleeping and "you know what." Using it often to read, watch TV, work, or anything else but the "big two" only makes it harder to fall asleep when the time comes.

Balance by "fixing your face." Your posture conveys everything about you—what you're thinking about, how self-assured you are, even your attitude toward whom you're with and what you're doing at that moment.

I remember seeing a replay of one of my earlier matches and my posture really conveyed how I felt. I hadn't been confident at all—and my body showed it. It was so obvious to me—and I'm sure my opponent and everyone else—that I was afraid and doubtful of what I could do. And from that day forward, I started reminding myself that even if I felt that way in the moment, I would never let it show.

I call it "fixing your face," and that means you always need to project the outcome that you want to happen. If that outcome is to be a leader, then you need to project that you're a leader. If it's to look confident, then you must project that you're confident. If you want to belong, you must project that you belong. And all that self-assurance starts with your eyes—which should convey that you have no fear by always making eye contact—and follows through in your posture.

You want your posture to look confident yet relaxed, not all stuffy and stiff. Pulling that off doesn't have to be that much work—it just means being *aware* of your posture every chance you get. At any given moment, your spine should be straight, shoulders back, head looking forward with your ears in line with your hips.

If that sounds like a lot of work, you don't have to overthink it too much. Whenever I'm aware of my posture, I tighten up my core muscles and imagine a string attached to my head that's being gently tugged upward. That may sound weird, but you'll be surprised at how just the thought of that crazy image will make you align yourself a little straighter than you were before. But in between those moments, by being smart about the positions you put your body through, you can improve your posture—and fix your face—even more, such as through these methods:

- If you sit often, you're putting stress on your joints and discs, as well as overstretching certain muscles that can pull your body out of alignment. Set a timer or make a point to get up and walk around for a few minutes every twenty minutes.
- Whenever you sit, continue to use the string trick, but keep your butt flat against the back of the chair and make sure your legs are bent at a ninety degree angle—you want your knees to be in line

with your hips. If they're not, put a box under your feet or adjust the chair.
- Position the chair (if possible) so that the armrests are at elbow height (that way, you won't have to bend forward to use them).

Balance by living for today—not just tomorrow. I've always found it funny how so many people think finding balance is something they'll eventually get around to doing once they're much older and have less to worry about. I mean, how many times have you heard someone say, "When I retire, I'll finally be able to do it all!"

It makes sense on paper. Without bosses to answer to, kids to clean up after, and all the other responsibilities that come with being an adult, you no longer have a thousand things to take on, which finally equals living a balanced life. But then again, I've also heard so many people say that, once they retired, they became bored.

That's just it. No one is too young to start living for today. Enjoying the moment, taking that trip, or having that experience in the *now* versus a *few years from now* is so important because what you're essentially doing is creating memories—and that's really what life is all about. And the longer you wait to create those memories, the less time you have to recall those memories over your lifetime. On top of that, even when you *think* you finally have enough time, you may find that your life is still out of balance because you lose purpose. You may no longer have the mobility and health for—or access to—the things, activities, events, people, etc., that genuinely bring you joy.

Should you plan for tomorrow? Absolutely. But should you put off everything until tomorrow? Absolutely not.

If it's something you could squeeze in, if it's a moment that you can create if you're honest with yourself, then seize it! Focus on what you *wish* you had more time for, ask yourself why you don't—and then figure out a way to make some time, even if it's just a little. It's finding these moments that will help you face other areas in your life more courageously and positively throughout the rest of your time. A few of my favorite tips:

- ***If you have a bucket list, start now.*** If you're waiting until you reach a certain age, place in your career, or the time when the kids have grown up, ask yourself what would happen if you started before that. Would it really be possible to do? If the answer is honestly yes, then stop waiting around and start living instead.

- ***Divide your dreams into how long they'll take you.*** Certain aspirations, like finally getting around to reading that book you've always been curious about or trying a painting class, aren't that much of a commitment, whereas changing your career or realizing your dream of writing a book may require a little more of your time. But having a sense of which dreams we can pull off more easily can propel us to do things we have put on the back burner.

CHAPTER 6

ENRICH

I've always believed that if something's too easy for you, then you're probably not growing or improving from it that much.

What I mean by that is this: While it's great to be consistent with making and maintaining healthier choices, if you simply "settle" for those choices, even if they are doing your body plenty of good in the moment, it's very easy to become bored, get stuck in place, or even slip backward when it comes to your progress.

Living your best life possible is all about moving forward instead of standing still. Even if you take what you're already doing right (eating certain healthy foods, getting enough exercise, making the right healthful choices for yourself, etc.) and merely improve on it just a tiny bit.

Think about it this way. It's like when the first affordable car—the Ford Model T—hit the streets in 1908. I'm sure back then, people were probably blown away to be able to sit behind a wheel instead of a horse and buggy to get around town. But imagine if those same people had just stayed content with that model. Today, you and I would be stuck driving cars with no air conditioning that could barely break 40 mph and—worse still—there would be no such thing as a Ferrari. You need to be mindful of all the different ways you could be boosting the smart decisions you're already making with your diet, your activities, and the things and people around you. In other words, even if you're happy with the way things are going, it's important to always bring in something new whenever possible. Besides, there's a risk of missing out by not enriching your life, because the next best thing for you might be right around the corner. But you'll never know it if you keep everything in your life exactly as it is.

Something else I have always felt strongly about is the importance of enriching others' lives along the way as well. When you support others and help them to move forward and grow, then you move forward and grow as well. When we do this, we enrich ourselves, the world around us, and the joy that's already in our lives. I'm talking about enriching anything and anyone, from those you care about most to perfect strangers, even causes or projects you feel a personal connection to. I'm talking about not just giving to charity but about contributing to your relationships and any mentors you have or have had along the way.

Enrich—The Right Way

I want you to think about how you can enrich the work you're doing and the people around you, but do so in thoughtful ways. Here are a few tips and tricks:

Don't treat small enhancements with any less respect. Some of the ways you'll learn how to enrich what you're already doing may seem small, but that doesn't make them any less important. Even the tiniest of changes can have a big impact. So instead of side-eyeing some of the suggestions, take them seriously if you want to maximize your results.

Don't tweak too soon. As excited as you might be about some of the changes you'll be making, you also need to be patient with them. It's important to let things breathe. So many of us expect instant results right from day one that if we don't see some sort of immediate change within ourselves, we either quit altogether—or suddenly feel the need to push ourselves even harder.

Being too impatient can cause some people to keep ratcheting up what they're already doing repeatedly until it's at a level that's not sustainable or fun anymore. That's why I want you to give any change you're making a minimum of a few weeks to see whether it's having an impact on your life.

Don't be afraid to explore other options. I promise you, with each healthful change you make along this journey, you're going to see a difference, whether in the short term or the long term. How big of a difference—and how quickly you'll see those results—is up to you and where you're presently at with your diet, activity level, and so on. But that doesn't mean you have to remain loyal to every enrichment you put in place.

The fun part about this section is that it's filled with a variety of different ways to enrich certain areas of your life—but none of them are written in stone. You can mix and match as many as you can handle, keep certain ones in place forever if you like them, or never try others if they just don't appeal to you. It's all about tailoring this to you—and enhancing what you're already doing so you STRIVE even further.

Enrich—Your Diet

Upgrading what you eat or drink is important, not only to bring more value to whatever smart nutritional choices you're already making or starting to make but also just to keep things fresh.

Face it, eating healthy can be boring, but it doesn't have to be. It just takes knowing what to add, take away, or try when the moment strikes.

Enrich by upgrading your water. Elevating the flavor of plain aqua is easy enough to do, but when you do it right, it can inspire you to drink all day long because you want to—not because you have to. I'm not a big fan of using artificial flavor enhancers as much as I believe in using all-natural fruits and vegetables, spices, and even extracts. All you need to do is fill up a pitcher with cold water, then infuse it by throwing in a few of the following (but remember to let it sit for at least a few hours before drinking ☺):

- **Fruits:** Apples, oranges, pineapples, pears, strawberries, raspberries, lemons, limes, blueberries, cherries, grapefruits, kiwis, or melons (any type).
- **Vegetables:** Cucumbers, celery, carrots, or jalapeno peppers.
- **Spices:** Sliced ginger, seedless vanilla beans, cinnamon sticks, cloves, sliced fennel bulbs, or cardamom pods.
- **Herbs and flowers (edible):** Dried hibiscus, rose petals, sage, lavender, cilantro, basil leaves, lemongrass, mint leaves, thyme, parsley, or rosemary sprigs.

> **Tip:** Think about buying two pitchers if you have room. That way you'll always have one to drink from today while the other one's busy infusing what you'll be drinking tomorrow.

Don't have room in your fridge (or need something a little more convenient)? Purchase a wide variety of extracts you would typically use in recipes—such as mint, almond, lemon, vanilla, or orange, for example—then try a drop or two in a glass of water. Or chop up a few peeled lemons, limes, or oranges (any fruit that's juicy), freeze them, then use them as ice cubes. Either can make plain water a lot more enticing without adding any extra calories or unwanted, unhealthy ingredients.

Enrich by spicing things up a bit. When most people need to boost the flavor of healthy foods, the usual go-tos tend to be condiments and sauces loaded with sugar, cholesterol, sodium, fat, calories, and a list of unpronounceable artificial ingredients. Instead, adding spices and herbs to foods that could use a little kick can satisfy your stomach without bringing any unhealthy baggage to the table.

Personally, I always use garlic, but I don't want you to have garlic breath to the point where people are staying away from you. Some of my favs are salts infused with flavors (I just got hooked on a raspberry salt that's incredible, for example) and different varieties of grindable peppercorns, like white, pink, and even Szechuan. But there are so many things you can add that bring not only the flavor (so you're more likely to enjoy the healthy foods you're choosing) but a few side perks in terms of nutritional benefits as well. Some of my favorite ways to enrich what I'm eating include:

- **Cardamom:** Packed with iron and manganese, this hot-sweet spice aids digestion, lowers blood pressure[1] and even protects you against bad bacteria.[2]
- **Cayenne pepper:** I love cayenne pepper because it contains capsaicin, a compound shown to alleviate aches and pains, to aid with circulation, and to possibly even improve vascular and metabolic health.[3]
- **Ceylon cinnamon:** Fortified with antioxidants including iron, calcium, and manganese, this also helps with insulin resistance and balancing your blood sugar.[4]

- **Cumin:** Helpful for controlling your blood pressure and killing bad bacteria, this spice also aids with digestion and fights inflammation.[5]
- **Curry Powder:** A mix of a variety of spices—including cardamom, cinnamon, and turmeric, among others—this powder is packed with antioxidants, fights inflammation, helps with digestion, and contains curcumin, which has been shown to help with digestion[6] and even destroy tumor cells.[7]
- **Garlic:** This is my favorite add-on and an immune system booster that fights cancer and contains allicin, a compound which has been shown to reduce your risk of stroke and heart disease.
- **Ginger:** This anti-inflammatory not only prevents nausea,[8] aids digestion, and helps your body absorb essential nutrients but it may even decrease your risk of cancer.[9]
- **Oregano:** This pizza topping favorite is also a powerful anti-inflammatory that goes after bad bacteria[10] and even suppresses cancer agents.[11]
- **Parsley:** This simple garnish contains flavonoids that may decrease your risk of cancer.[12]
- **Rosemary:** Not only does this fragrant anti-inflammatory spice help improve memory but it also has antibacterial properties in addition to suppressing cancer in the breast, colon, liver, and stomach.[13]
- **Sweet Basil:** It doesn't just smell incredible, but it's also an anti-inflammatory[14] teeming with vitamin A, vitamin K, lutein, potassium, and calcium.
- **Thyme:** This tasty spice has vitamins, minerals, and an antimicrobial compound—thymol—a natural anticarcinogen.[15]
- **Turmeric:** Beyond having antioxidant and anti-inflammatory benefits, this spice may also help prevent memory loss, as well as reverse certain symptoms related to obesity including hyperglycemia, hyperlipidemia, and insulin resistance.[16]

To be honest, unless you're allergic to a particular herb or spice, you can't go wrong with choosing any type (celery seed, coriander, dill, sage, paprika, tarragon, fennel, you name it). But to get the most out of any of them, consider the following:

Buy them whole whenever possible. They last longer and taste better than ground versions, but you'll need either a mortar and pestle or spice grinder to prepare them when you want them.

Put them someplace dark and dry. Resist having them conveniently sitting out in your kitchen. Store them in airtight containers away from light, heat, or moisture, which can change how they taste.

Check the expiration date. Herbs and spices are like a new car. They start depreciating the moment you drive them off the lot, losing their flavor and becoming less potent. Keep them for a year, then kick them to the curb.

If buying fresh, have a game plan. Nothing beats basil, cilantro, or other herbs fresh from the garden, but they can spoil quickly. If you're going to use them in a few days, either cut the stems and place them in a glass of water in your refrigerator, or if they're just leaves that can't be snipped, put them in an open plastic bag inside your crisper drawer.

Enrich by rethinking what you pick. Chances are, even though you'll be balancing your diet in different ways as you STRIVE, you're most likely still turning to a lot of your favorite foods and meals. But if you arm yourself with a few simple tricks, you could cleverly reduce the unwanted calories, unhealthy fat, and unnatural ingredients you're taking in whenever you turn to your go-to foods. Before your next meal or snack, give some thought to these effortless ways to enrich them without calling attention to yourself.

Do a leg count. If you're ever given a choice between different types of meats, stick with whichever animal has the least number of legs. It's not 100 percent foolproof (depending on the cut or how it's cooked), but the order of what's healthiest typically goes fish (no legs), poultry (two legs), then pork or beef (four legs). The fewer legs your meal once had, the less fat and low-density lipoprotein (LDL) cholesterol you'll be eating along with it.

Go backward from the good stuff. Instead of randomly eating what's on your plate or starting with what you love, reverse the order so you start with the healthiest and/or least caloric thing—then work up from there. If you don't clear your plate, chances are you'll be just as full as you would have been, but you'll have eaten fewer calories. Plus, it guarantees you won't be leaving behind what's probably the most nutritious thing on your plate.

Reconsider what's in your hands. Something as simple as placing your spoon or fork down between bites can reduce the urge to eat more than necessary. Better still, pick up a pair of chopsticks instead (no matter what type of food you're eating). They may be annoying to grab certain foods with, but that's the whole point! You'll be left with no choice but to eat more slowly (and in smaller portions) than usual.

Reach for what's ready to rot first. Gross, right? Actually, it's not. I'm not talking about eating whatever's going bad. I'm saying that if you have to choose one food over another and can't decide between the two, pick the one that's more perishable. The more likely something is to last, the more artificial ingredients and preservatives it probably contains. Picking the food more likely to spoil means you're probably choosing something that's healthier for you.

Rotate to avoid a food rut. It's a simple fact that every food has a unique combination of vitamins and minerals. Sticking with your favorites too often, even if they're healthy for you, could leave you deficient in whatever nutrients those particular foods lack. To give yourself a better shot at getting a more complete balance of vitamins and minerals, put a little more space between your favorite go-to meals than you typically do to allow other foods with different nutrient ratios to sneak in there.

Look for a better ratio. The next time you find yourself torn between two types of foods, turn them both over, look at the ingredient list, then pick the one with less. Healthier foods tend to have fewer ingredients (for example, when was the last time you saw more than one ingredient listed on a bag of oranges?), but if you're still not sure (or it's a tie), see which one has the most ingredients you don't recognize. Anything unrecognizable or unpronounceable is most likely artificial and something you shouldn't be putting into your body anyway.

Jump through hoops for the bad stuff. Ninety percent of the time, we've got to be good. But then there's the other 10 percent where we get to be a little bad. You're going to get that craving for something delicious you know isn't good for you, but you're going to eat it anyway. When that happens, at least do yourself a favor and try to make it a little more difficult by:

- *Making it yourself.* For example, when I'm craving French fries, I'll cut up a potato, put some seasonings on it, bake it, and I'm good to go. But even if you can't find a healthier alternative to cook or bake, doing it yourself keeps you more accountable for what you're about to eat.

- *Making it a road trip.* If it's a fast food or something you have to pick up, put some distance between you and your appetite by picking a restaurant that's farther away than closer.

- *Making it hard to reach.* Honestly, put whatever junk food tempts you someplace where it takes a lot of effort to get it. The trunk of your car, up in a high cabinet that takes a stepladder to reach it, down in your basement—somewhere that's not easy to get to every time you feel like grabbing a handful of it.

Enrich by rethinking your drinks. It's not only a little too easy to drink a lot of extra calories you don't really need when choosing certain beverages (such as soda, fruit juice, and coffee) but many drinks also tend to be loaded in sugar and artificial ingredients that can negatively affect your overall health. But if you're a little wiser with what you pour yourself, it can do your body a world of good. Here are a few ways to enrich what you drink by pulling back on what's keeping you from moving forward.

Coffee: It actually contains zero calories, but good luck finding many people who drink it that way. It's the extra stuff you must watch out for, which is why I like to *spoon* in—not *pour* in— whatever I flavor it with. That way, you can truly see how many calories you're adding as you go. On average:

Skim milk (one tbsp.): five calories
Whole milk (one tbsp.): ten calories
Sugar (one tsp.): sixteen calories

Half-and-half (one tbsp.): twenty calories
Agave nectar (one tsp.): twenty calories
Liquid concentrate creamers (one tbsp.): average thirty-five calories
Heavy whipping cream (one tbsp.): fifty-plus calories
Raw honey (one tbsp.): sixty calories

Better still, try to pick something that gives something back. Sure, raw honey has a lot of calories, but it's also packed with enzymes and nutrients, including potassium, calcium, iron, and all the B-complex vitamins. (**Tip:** The darker it is, the more antioxidants it has, so pick a bottle you can't see through.)[17]

Another way to enrich your coffee is to not have that second cup in the first place. For some, it's just out of habit to have more than one. Instead, try switching it out with a different warm drink in the same cup (wash it first obviously), such as chai tea, green or black tea, steeped ginger, hot cacao, or just hot water with a little lemon.

Soda: Lacking anything nutritious, soda isn't just empty calories but it also raises your blood sugar and blood pressure, as well as increases your risk of kidney damage, diabetes, and heart disease. And the no- to low-calorie varieties? They're no better, since the artificial sweeteners found in most diet drinks (like saccharin, aspartame, and sucralose) are known neurotoxins and carcinogens.

Ask yourself: Is sparing yourself a hundred-plus calories a soda worth increasing your risk of a wide variety of health issues, including fibromyalgia, multiple sclerosis, lymphoma, Alzheimer's, you name it? Right, I didn't think so. Instead, try a sugar-free, all-natural carbonated water (sweetened with either stevia or monk fruit) to satisfy your sweet tooth.

Alcohol: I'd be a hypocrite if I said stay away from alcohol. I'll have periods when I will drink and have wine nights, but I keep it under control. Part of it is for vanity, but the other reason is for my health, which is why it's important to realize how alcohol affects your body, even in the short term.

I wish I could drink more often than I do because I love my wines, and for a lot of people, alcohol can be enjoyable with a good meal, when you're out with friends, watching a movie or game, and all that. But I temper it because I also understand how, when you drink alcohol, your liver (the organ responsible for filtering and storing nutrients) processes more slowly, making it harder to distribute whatever important nutrients you've already eaten throughout your body where they're needed. It's also seven calories per gram (that has zero nutritional value whatsoever), plus it raises your blood sugar, spiking your insulin levels, which causes your body to store some of those extra useless calories as body fat.

Just the same, when you do choose to drink, you have a few wiser choices you could turn to:

Red wine: It's a top choice because it's high in resveratrol, an antioxidant found in grapes, cranberries, blueberries, and other foods that's been proven to lower bad cholesterol, blood pressure, and inflammation. It also can keep your blood vessels healthy and can even slow down tumor growth.[18]

Anything dark: The darker-colored versions of alcohol—like a stout or whiskey—tend to have more antioxidants and polyphenols (plant-based micronutrients that help lower your risk of heart disease, diabetes, and cancer, and can activate your immune system to fight off infection and disease).

Any drink in general: If you're thirsty and plain old water won't do, at least take a moment and pause before you sip away on your first choice of drink. In fact, challenge yourself to "downgrade" that chosen drink with something that beats it. Using this table of common drinks listed from calorically high to low, find whatever you're about to drink, then consider a beverage a few spots below it. So long as it's one that's nutritious, you'll be taking in fewer calories for the same amount of liquid.

Drink	Serving Size (ounces)	Average Calories
Chocolate milk (whole)	12	300–320
Chocolate milk (1 percent)	12	230–240
Grape juice	12	225
Milk (whole)	12	220
Café latte with whole milk	12	205
Cranberry juice cocktail	12	200
Pineapple juice (canned)	12	200
Pomegranate juice	12	200
Milk (2 percent)	12	180
Orange juice	12	170–225
Apple juice (unsweetened)	12	170
Cranberry juice (unsweetened)	12	165
Milk (1 percent)	12	155
Beer (regular)	12	150
Carrot juice	12	150
Grapefruit juice (pink/white)	12	130–145
Soda (regular)	12	120–190
Wine (red/white)	5	120–125
Milk (skim)	12	120
Cappuccino with whole milk	12	110
Alcohol (eighty-proof rum, vodka, whiskey, gin)	1.5	100
Caffe latte with skim milk	12	100
Beer (light)	12	100
V8 vegetable juice	12	75
Coconut water	12	60–70

Tomato juice	12	60–70
Coffee with two tbsps. half-and-half	12	60
Coffee with two tbsps. milk (1 percent or skim)	12	25
Diet soda	12	0–10
Coffee (black)	12	0–5
Unsweetened tea	12	0–5
Green tea (bagged/loose)	12	0
Seltzer, sparkling, tap, or mineral water	12	0

Enrich by covering your nutrient bases. Although I believe getting nutrients directly from food is optimal, relying solely on food alone for your nutrients could leave you nutritionally deficient. Do I believe in supplementation to enrich your diet? Yes, but most lifestyle books just rattle off a list of vitamins and minerals they want you to take and leave it at that. That's not how it works. Our bodies have different needs for themselves, just like we all have different goals for ourselves. And while I believe in taking a daily multivitamin, I don't believe people should just take it as a one-and-done catchall.

That's why, if you're serious about trying supplementation to fill in the gaps, take a trip to your doctor and get blood work to find out specifically what vitamins and minerals you may be lacking in. That should be your starting place, because even though there are so many amazing things to take, certain ones may not be necessary for you (and will be a waste of money) while others might be vital for your health.

For example, I take a vitamin D supplement along with zinc, magnesium, and iron (among others), but that's what my body needs. Once you know what yours does, all I ask is that you:

- *Buy from the right companies.* If you see the words USDA Organic, GMP Quality, or Non-GMO Project Verified on the package, the product has been vetted by a reputable third party to make sure what you're buying is exactly what it claims it is.

- **Stick with organic when possible.** Because many herbal supplements are less likely to have third-party verification, buying organic ensures that you're getting herbs that are free of pesticides. Credible companies often provide information on where their raw ingredients come from, but look for the USDA Organic certification seal.
- **Take them at the right times.** Ideally, taking a multivitamin first thing in the morning with breakfast will guarantee you don't forget taking it later in the day. However, if you need to supplement a specific vitamin or mineral for some reason, pay close attention to how it may be best absorbed. For example, taking any of the eight B vitamins on an empty stomach is thought to be more effective, while fat-soluble vitamins, such as vitamin A, are best taken with a meal containing fats.

Enrich—Your Activities

It doesn't matter what activities or exercises you turn to in order to get fit, or that you might love to do them more than anything. Eventually, you're going to have to add a little extra to whatever you choose to do to see more results and beat boredom to the punch—especially if your plan is to stay fit for life.

Enrich by changing things up often. If you want to see results from exercise—I mean continual results—you need to keep your body constantly challenged with routines that confuse your muscles before they become a little too comfortable. What do I mean by that? It works like this: Start a new exercise routine and your muscles work overtime because you're hitting them with a combination of movements and tempos they're not familiar with. Because of that lack of familiarity, they work a lot harder—and burn a lot more calories—to get the job done.

But stick with the same workout for too long, and not only are you more likely to become bored with it and hate it but your body quickly begins to adapt to it. After that, it doesn't take long for your body to figure out how to pull off the same workout using less effort and fewer calories.

To make matters worse, every workout routine puts a unique combination of stress on muscle fibers, joints, tendons, and other areas of your body. The longer you stick with the same program, the greater your risk of injury from overusing certain areas (by never giving them a break) and of creating muscular imbalances that could impact your performance.

If all that sounds scary (and changing workouts and exercises around sounds like way too much work), don't worry about it. By making just the slightest of changes to your routine, you can keep your body out of its comfort zone—and continuously burn calories and build lean muscle as a result. Making sure your muscles stay interested enough to evolve only takes tweaking any of a variety of factors (so long as you're fit enough to do it):

- **The tempo:** Instead of raising and lowering the weights (or yourself, if doing a body-weight exercise) at a pace of two seconds up/two seconds down, try speeding up the tempo (one second up/one second down), slowing it down (three-plus seconds up/three-plus seconds down), or even alternating the tempo (three-plus seconds down/one second up, for example).
- **The rest time:** Traditionally, resting between sixty to ninety seconds between exercises is fine. But you could always reduce that time to less than sixty seconds (to forty-five, thirty, or fifteen seconds, for instance) or forget about resting in between altogether.
- **The number of reps:** As I mentioned in the "Balance" chapter, doing eight to twelve repetitions of an exercise might be standard,

but you can always play with those numbers and do fewer (six to eight, four to six, etc.) or more (fifteen to twenty or twenty to twenty-five, for example), so long as you're choosing a weight that's heavy enough to exhaust your muscles within whatever number of reps decide on.

- **The number of sets:** Doing two to four sets of an exercise is recommended, but there's nothing stopping you from doing as little as one set or as many as ten occasionally, just to shock your body. So long as you're challenging your muscles without overtaxing them, feel free to experiment.
- **The exercises:** Try taking the routine you're currently doing and just do the exercises out of order. You'll be exhausting certain muscle fibers sooner than they're used to, which can make the routine feel entirely different to your muscles.
- **The whole thing:** Finally, say good-bye to your workout after four to six weeks no matter how much you love it. Don't wait until you quit being active altogether to change your routine.

Enrich by rethinking your "in-activity." You don't spend every waking minute of your life in the gym, do you? And if you do, do you really want to?

The point is, sure, you burn calories by exercising, but you can't exercise all the time—that's overkill and not healthy for you in the first place. But you can still burn more calories during all those moments when you're literally just sitting or standing around. It just takes a little creativity on your part:

Whenever you're standing . . .

- Bend your left knee slightly, then raise your right foot about an inch off the ground—either in front of yourself or behind you— then balance yourself that way for as long as you comfortably can. Then switch positions (bending your right knee slightly and raising your left foot) and repeat. Stand back up, rest for fifteen to thirty seconds, and repeat eight to ten times.

- Bend both knees and squat about an inch or so (just enough so that your legs aren't in a locked position but not so much that it's noticeable if you are feeling self-conscious), then hold that position for as long as you comfortably can. Stand back up, rest for fifteen to thirty seconds, and repeat eight to ten times.

Whenever you're sitting . . .

- Keeping your back straight and your core muscles tight, plant your feet slightly wider than shoulder-width apart, then gently push your heels into the floor. You shouldn't really move, but you'll feel all the muscles throughout your legs from your heels to your butt engaged. Hold that pose for as long as you comfortably can, relax, then repeat eight to ten times.
- Fidget as much as possible (meaning frequently reposition yourself in your seat, tap your toes, shake your legs, etc.). You may feel silly, but fidgeting has been shown to burn up to 350 extra calories a day.

Note: None of these "inconspicuous" exercises are intense enough that they should interfere with your workouts, your sport, or any other activity that may require your muscles to be primed and ready. But that doesn't mean you can't overdo it if you're literally trying them all day long. That said, if you're thinking of incorporating some or all of these into your day, start slowly and try them two to three times daily, then see if they impact your performance in your workouts or other activities. If they don't, slowly increase how many times you do them each day.

Enrich by fueling your workouts. Right before you exercise (between thirty to sixty minutes prior), I want you to have a small snack (around a few hundred calories at the most). Then, once you're done exercising (between thirty to sixty minutes afterward), I want you to have another small snack (again, just a few hundred calories' worth).

Eating before and after you exercise might feel counterproductive, especially if one of your goals is weight loss. However, there's a lot of science that supports how having the right foods both before and after you work out can help you see more results—including burning more fat.

It works like this: Is it true that working out on an empty stomach leaves your body little choice but to burn more body fat as energy? Definitely, but—and only you can answer this about yourself—if exercising that way typically leaves you feeling sluggish, less energized, or lightheaded, then you might be keeping yourself from working out with as much intensity. Or worse, you could quit before the workout's over because you've run out of steam. Having a snack prior can give you enough fuel to prevent that from happening.

Why would you want to eat something immediately afterward then? That's easy—you're doing it for two important reasons:

1. Right after you exercise, one of your body's immediate goals is to refill its glycogen, the carbohydrates it stores inside your muscles and liver that it uses for energy (along with body fat). To do that, it turns to food, but if there's nothing in your stomach, it's left with little choice but to break down your muscles instead.

2. On days that you do some type of resistance training, your body starts searching for amino acids immediately afterward to rebuild your muscles. If you don't eat anything, it pauses that process, preventing your muscles from recovering as quickly from your workouts.

Do I have to eat before? Like I said, it's up to you. If you don't notice a difference in your performance going into your workouts with an empty belly versus having a small snack, then that's fine.

What if I typically exercise right before (or after) breakfast, lunch, or dinner? In that case, you could split up your meal into two portions. Have a smaller portion thirty to sixty minutes before you work out, then eat the rest of your meal immediately after you're done exercising.

Can I eat right before I work out? You could, but keep in mind that digesting food takes energy—energy that could be used to fuel your workout instead of breaking down what's in your stomach. But if you have no choice on certain days, that's fine.

What's the best kind of "snack"? If you need a pre-workout snack for a quick energy boost, a mix of fast-burning simple and complex carbohydrates works best. If you have protein, that's fine, but stay away from fats (which take longer to digest). Post-workout, eating a mix of protein and carbohydrates to give your body what it needs to rebuild and restore is your smartest bet.

Need a few creative ideas that are just the right number of calories and macronutrients? Try the following on for size:

Pre-workout

- One slice of whole-wheat bread with a piece of fruit.
- A small bowl of oatmeal or whole-grain cereal with a few berries or raisins.
- A whole-grain fig bar.
- A handful of dried fruit.

Post-workout

- One glass of chocolate milk.
- A half of a banana and one to two tablespoons of all-natural almond or peanut butter.

- A piece of fresh fruit with one or two small hard-boiled eggs.
- A half cup of cottage cheese with chopped-up fruit thrown on top.
- A serving of plain Greek yogurt mixed with a handful of chopped almonds, berries, or granola.
- A serving of tuna salad with a few whole-grain crackers.

Enrich—Who and What's Around You

Wanting a better life is a worthwhile goal, but if you're just doing things for yourself, then your life—no matter how fulfilling you think it might be—is way too small. It's as simple as that. Your life should always be greater than you—and greater than one person—because if you only have yourself, you have a number that's never going to multiply.

That's one times zero.

But when you're able to help other people, then your life becomes greater than yourself. It becomes bigger and more fulfilling than you will ever accomplish on your own, and it's only through helping others achieve *their* best life possible that you'll achieve your best life possible.

So how can you do that? Easy. It's about being of service to others by making a part of your day thinking, "How can I help those around me today—even beyond my friends and family?" It really doesn't take a lot to make a big impact in someone else's life, but it does require some form of support, time, or encouragement on your part.

Enrich by thanking five people today. My dad was always very serious and worked hard, so he expected the same from anyone who helped my sister and me—coaches, physical therapists, you name it. Whenever he would see those same traits in others, he was always appreciative and super grateful, constantly saying things like, "Thank you for being here," or "You're doing an amazing job," to everyone in a genuine, meaningful way. He had this way of making people feel great about who they were and what they did. That's behavior I've tried to model as well, because just saying "thank you"—especially when it's unprompted and unexpected—is both super powerful and incredibly meaningful.

Think about the last time someone said "thank you" to you. It doesn't matter what you did to earn it. All I care about is how it made you feel. Pretty nice, right? Maybe you didn't feel amazing for hours afterward, but in that moment, being thanked meant being acknowledged for whatever it was you did. Knowing how powerful that phrase is to you when it's aimed in your direction, it's important to remember that you have the power to make somebody feel like that too.

Two words—thank you—are all it takes to remind someone how they did something good. Two words to make someone feel a little prouder of themselves, so much so that they might want to repeat that kind act over and over again.

It doesn't have to be for something someone just did for you. In fact, thanking somebody for something they did for you in the past can have more value because it means you really thought about them in that moment. And you don't even have to thank someone for something they did directly for you. Thanking anyone in your community for doing a great job—a teacher, a hospital worker, a coach, etc.—also counts. You may not have an impact on everybody, but if you thank five people today, I guarantee at least one of them will be moved by your words of kindness.

Enrich by celebrating someone's victories as if they're your own. When someone succeeds at something, even if you're genuinely happy for them, how much time do you spend focusing on their achievements? What I mean is, instead of just listening to them, nodding, and recognizing what they've done, do you make the effort to ask them to go into more detail about how they accomplished it?

The next time someone tells you they succeeded at something—maybe they finished a race, got a promotion at work, earned their *insert college degree of choice here*, whatever it might be—don't just listen, but tell them how proud you are of them, then dare to dig deeper. I'm talking about asking more thoughtful questions beyond the typical "How long did it take you?" such as:

- What motivated you to want to do that?
- What was the most difficult obstacle to overcome—and what was the easiest?
- What steps did you take to reach your goal?
- What's the next goal you have for yourself to keep that momentum going?

What I love about doing this is that it not only motivates that person but their answers may end up motivating you. By diving deeper into what they're proud of, you might walk away with a better game plan to tackle that same task or some tips and tricks that might work with something else you're going through now. But at the very least, you've shown that person genuine interest in what interests them, and that can lead to that person being there for you when it's your turn to succeed.

Enrich by offering up your talents. Time is precious, and most days, we only have a limited number of hours to spread any sort of love to others. So how can you make the biggest impact with whatever time you have to give?

In my experience, it's about playing to your strengths and what you're enthusiastic about. What I mean by that is this: When possible, find some way to help others that you're equally excited about. Because in my experience, being passionate about what you're planning on sharing with others is so very important when you're in that "giving" zone.

For example, three of my greatest passions are sports (obviously!), wellness, and the arts. They're areas where I not only feel I have a lot to share but many seem curious to pick my brain about. So, whenever I offer pointers on any of the above, not only do others get excited because they're moving forward, but I'm just as jazzed because I'm talking from a place of self-assurance and happiness.

I don't know what you're good at, but I do know that everybody is good at something—and is probably that way because they're passionate about it. So, consider what you're at least a little better than someone at. (Maybe it's an activity, a sport, gardening, changing your car's oil—it really doesn't matter!) You don't have to be an expert on whatever it is. You just have to be willing to share those passions with others when they ask, or if they're not the type to ask, be ready to lend a helpful hand whenever you see someone in need of what you know.

The best part about it is that sharing your passions with others may indirectly help someone find theirs as well. For example, what sparked my interest in the arts was watching my mom sew when I was a kid. I just couldn't get enough of it, and I still wish I had all the time in the world to just sew and make clothes all day, but that was my first exposure to art of any kind.

After that, I realized how much I absolutely loved the arts and got involved in many kinds of artistic pursuits, exposing myself to every type I could. Industrial design and architecture, graphic design, sculpture, photography—it didn't matter what it was because I loved learning about and being around all of it. Even things that might seem a little dry to some are exciting for me. In fact, whenever I finally get to see pieces of art I've only read about or seen online, I get so excited I'm like, "Agh! This! This is a moment!" But at a certain point, I knew there were only so many hours in a day, and I chose to focus on interior design and fine art. I got my degree, and now I'm the CEO of my own interior design firm, V Starr Interiors. All because someone—my mom—shared her talents with me.

Enrich by making your day about someone else. In this book, I'm asking you to pay a lot of attention to different aspects of your life all day long, but now it's time to flip the script. Instead of just doing things for yourself, I want you to choose anyone in your life and make the day about them.

You can give them a heads-up beforehand so they're not too surprised when you make yourself available out of left field, but make sure they understand you're ready to assist them with anything they need that day. No reason given. Not because it's their birthday or anything special. No, the only reason you're doing it is because they're a friend.

Think about it this way: We're always juggling a million things, but what if a friend came up to you and offered the same help out of nowhere? Told you that they were ready to tackle some of the tasks, jobs, or errands you had on your plate at that moment? How good would that feel?

That's the point of enriching somebody this way as often as possible. Because even if you didn't have that much going on—because let's face it, some days we're not always stressed out or stretched thin—wouldn't it be nice to know there's somebody out there who would even consider doing that for you? That's the same feeling you're going to bring to that person, enriching them by either easing their anxiety by dividing their workload, or reminding them somebody is watching out for them.

Enrich—Yourself

Look up the word *enrich* in the dictionary, and you'll find a slew of synonyms like *upgrade, elevate,* and *enhance,* just to name a few. That being the case, everything in this book is "enriching you" to some degree. Improving your diet, exercising more, putting serious thought into the connections you have with others—all these initiatives will come together and upgrade, elevate, and enhance you to some degree.

However, there's always other areas related to ourselves that could use a little more attention. Areas that may not be as top of mind, but when you take the time to address them, they can build upon everything else you're setting in motion, making it easier to steer yourself toward your best life possible.

Enrich by organizing *some* of your stuff. For me, an organized environment helps me be more effective and feel more clear-headed. An environment that's unorganized? Well, that's chaos for me, and I honestly can't think straight. That's why keeping my workspace clean—or any area where I'm trying to accomplish something positive for myself, like the gym, my kitchen, you name it—is something I always strive for.

Now, am I a master at it? Nope, and keeping all those spaces orderly all the time is something I haven't quite achieved yet and may never pull off. But as impossible as it may be to sort out everything, keeping at least *one thing* under control—even if it's only for a little while—can go a long way toward lessening your stress levels and improving your overall health.

Could I tell you how to organize yourself? Everyone's different, and I don't know which areas of your life are more chaotic than others. All I will say is this—look for the places in your life where you find yourself:

- Wasting time looking for what you need.
- Forgetting to do things that you should've remembered.
- Falling behind from where you thought you would be.
- Feeling more frustrated than fulfilled.

If that means needing to organize your desk one week, getting a handle on your work schedule the next, or taking control of your closet after that, attack whatever feels the most cluttered or disorganized in the moment.

Enrich by stepping up your sleep habits. Even if you're getting enough z's like I suggested in the "Balance" chapter, that doesn't mean you can't improve upon how you spend one-third of your day.

Position yourself as perfectly as possible. A whole host of problems can occur when you don't consider how your body's positioned, such as sleep apnea, heartburn, back pain, headaches, neck pain, muscle cramping, fatigue, and so many other health-related issues. But you can minimize your risk of any of the above by supporting your body the right way prior to falling asleep.

- *Side sleeper?* Start by bending your knees, then placing a pillow between them. (This keeps your spine and hips level to each other.)

- *Stomach sleeper?* Start by tucking a pillow underneath your stomach and hips to take pressure off your lower back by straightening out your spine.

- *Back sleeper?* Start with a rolled-up towel (or small pillow) underneath the small of your lower back, as well as a pillow directly underneath your knees.

Only wash your face with warm water. Using cold water to take makeup off or just feel fresh prior to bedtime can sometimes make you more alert.

Consider what wafts around you. Certain smells have been shown to lower stress and induce sleep more than others, so try diffusing or applying (when appropriate) any of the following scents: cedarwood, chamomile, jasmine, lavender, valerian, vanilla, ylang ylang, or any scent that you notice calms you down.

Reconsider your habits before bedtime. There are a few things you may want to stop doing as early as late afternoon when possible (up to six hours prior to bedtime) because of how they impact the quality of your sleep:

- Alcohol (even though it can make you sleepy) actually prevents restorative REM sleep and has been shown to potentially cause insomnia and sleep apnea.

- Nicotine, as well as caffeine from a variety of different sources (coffee, soda, certain types of tea—such as green, white, and black—chocolate, and certain caffeine-infused pain relievers, including Motrin and Excedrin), quickly overstimulates your nervous system and can make falling asleep much more difficult.

- Exercising right before bedtime may tire you out, but for some people, working out (or being active) prior to heading to bed can cause them to feel more energized and alert after they've elevated their heart rate.

Enrich by turning away from toxins. What you put on your body, what you clean your house with, what you expose your food to all create the potential to come into contact with toxins all around you.

Trying to avoid **every single one** of them **all** at the same time—well, good luck with that. To make matters worse, we all have certain things we may love—beauty products, that favorite water bottle, that frying pan you never have to work hard to clean—that may have a few "bad for you" toxins in them. But that doesn't mean you shouldn't try to find a win as often as possible using products free of as many toxins as possible. Try challenging yourself by spending the day doing your best—and doing your homework—to avoid contact with anything that could be exposing yourself to toxins, then find a healthier solution. Just a few considerations include:

- Avoid white coffee filters, paper towels, and other paper products (which are typically turned white using chlorine) and opt for brown versions.
- Pass on nonstick cookware coated with Teflon or other chemical substances and switch to ceramic, glass, cast iron, or stainless steel instead.
- Only clean with products labeled nontoxic, noncarcinogenic, nonpetroleum based, ammonia-free, biodegradable, or free of perfumes or dyes.
- Steer clear of eating seafood known to have high amounts of mercury, such as tuna, species of mackerel, swordfish, and orange roughy. If you need your fish, go with choices with the least amount of mercury, such as catfish, flounder, haddock, salmon, or tilapia.
- Don't store or reheat your food in plastic containers (use glass or ceramic instead).
- Switch your plastic water bottle for one lined with ceramic or stainless steel (not regular steel or aluminum).

Enrich by rewarding yourself the right way. Am I a big believer in rewarding yourself for a job well done? Sure I am. And as you hit certain goals as you STRIVE, who am I to stand in the way of you pampering yourself occasionally for crossing certain finish lines—whether that's after finally mastering a certain exercise, running your first 5K, or improving a particular health score. But how you spoil yourself can decide whether you keep moving forward or fall back.

Most people I know—and yes, I'm equally guilty, although not as much anymore—like to reward themselves with the unhealthiest meal imaginable after nailing a certain health goal. Would I stop you from chowing down on one bad meal if that's what kept you motivated to stay strong with your diet choices for the week? No, but it's sort of counterproductive, isn't it? All I'm suggesting are a few more creative (and healthier) ways to indulge yourself, such as:

- **Give yourself a needle mover:** New workout shoes, an Apple gift card (so you can buy inspirational music to work out to), a session with a personal trainer, a one-week gym membership somewhere else—think about something that might encourage you to exercise even more.

- **Give yourself a guilty pleasure:** Think of something you typically feel silly buying or doing for yourself for whatever reason—downloading a game app, binge-watching an entertaining show, buying a romance novel—then do it (but skip the guilt because you deserve it!).

- **Give yourself a beauty booster:** A trip to the nail or hair salon, new lipstick, a wax. Whatever would bring out even more of what makes you beautiful counts.

- **Give yourself a break:** Whether it's a spa visit, a day at the beach, or making a deal with your family to have an afternoon to yourself, think about what would really relax you if you had time, then make the time once you realize your goals.

CHAPTER 7

SOOTHE

Most people never recognize the importance of soothing themselves until it's too late. So many put all their energy into pushing themselves forward that they never make the time to place as much effort into, well—not pushing themselves.

Throughout my life, my mom always encouraged me to give myself enough downtime, which for me was—and still is—a very hard thing to do. Time and time again, she would say that if I didn't rest when necessary, my body would never have the chance to heal and that would only set me up for failure later on. I would be more likely to injure myself, get sick because I was too run-down, or be susceptible to all sorts of things that could keep me from STRIVING forward.

Whether it's not finding enough minutes in the day or plain stubborn pride thinking that whatever doesn't kill you makes you stronger, I (like I'm sure most people) will admit that I've been guilty of both. But I really had to learn the importance of giving my body a break the hard way when I was first diagnosed with Sjögren's syndrome.

As an athlete, I already knew how to dial things down at certain times to prevent overtraining and injury, but dealing with Sjögren's was entirely different. I had to consider every aspect of where stress can come from, not just from physical activity but what I ate, my surroundings, how I spent my free time, and even whom I chose to hang with. I had to relearn that just because I didn't *feel* stressed or sore most days didn't mean I wasn't always in desperate need of taking enough time to heal.

Since that time, following a raw vegan diet has definitely relieved some of the symptoms that come with Sjögren's, including fatigue, joint pain, and digestive issues. My diet helped me truly understand why it's so important to consider what we put into our bodies. But it's just as important to consider how we think. It's about learning how to control your mind and even turn it off when necessary to achieve a more restful and healing state.

There are so many ways you can self-soothe and heal your mind and body inside and out, from rethinking your consumption of certain things (such as fiber, alcohol, and meat), smart supplementation, adding the right nutrients to your diet, applying therapeutic methods (exercises, stretches, and massage), relying on meditation, as well as learning smarter ways to relieve anxiety and stress. All the above can help your mind and body recharge and recover quickly and easily. It honestly doesn't take that much to put yourself in a constant state of healing. It just takes spending a little time soothing certain areas of your life on a regular basis.

Soothe—The Right Way

Soothing may sound easy, but don't let the word fool you. Giving yourself the right recovery tools still requires a smart approach and the best sense of your body to minimize soreness, lessen fatigue, and make you more injury resistant. Here's what you need to remember to help accelerate the healing process every time you soothe:

Don't wait until something aches. Some of the soothing techniques in this section are methods that many people turn to *after* the fact. You might believe that soothing is only something you turn to during certain moments, such as right after intense exercise or after an injury.

Maybe you've been guilty of this as well. Have you ever stretched a muscle only after it felt tight? Went to bed early to get a decent sleep only after feeling exhausted from too many back-to-back nights of burning the midnight oil? Thought about meditation only because you were desperately trying to calm your mind after a hectic day? I thought so, because you're not alone.

But when you soothe yourself every day in as many ways as possible, you keep yourself in a constant state of healing. That means you won't experience aches and pains as often because you're already taking care of certain body parts before they become a problem. You never find yourself overly tired because you never let yourself get sleep deprived as frequently. You're never scrambling to ease your thoughts because your thoughts are already in a much calmer place.

Don't assume more is better. It's only natural to think that if something's good for you, then the more frequently you do it, the more results you'll see. But just like we can overdo it with exercise, work, or other areas of our lives by sometimes losing ourselves and pushing ourselves too hard, soothing works the exact same way.

The easiest example I can throw at you is rest. Is it important to give your body time off after exercise in order to let it heal? Absolutely. Is it smart to get plenty of sleep every night? Can't argue with that. But if you sat around for months giving yourself plenty of downtime and slept fourteen hours a night, what do you think would happen to your body? Like I said, too much of a good thing can be a bad thing—so stick with whatever is prescribed in the section.

Soothe—Your Diet

O nce you begin balancing and enriching your diet on a regular basis, you'll already be on your way to improving your health by soothing your body from the inside out. But why stop there? A lot of healthy foods have other healing properties to take advantage of that ease inflammation, strip away stress and anxiety, and promote better digestion. Try any of the following, or just pick and choose certain foods to add to whatever you're presently eating. Either way, you'll be soothing your body from the inside out.

Soothe your pH levels. Personally, I lean toward a plant-based alkaline diet, which basically means I balance my body's pH level by replacing or limiting acid-forming foods and eating more alkaline foods.

The theory is that certain foods cause your body to produce harmful acid. It's believed that certain types of cancer thrive in an acidic environment, but through eating certain foods, you can change your body's pH level (its acid level) and lower your cancer risk in addition to improving your health in other ways.

Now, do I believe all the science behind it? Am I strict with it? All I can say is, for me, I really notice a true difference when I keep my body more alkaline by eating an eighty-to-twenty ratio whenever I can. Meaning, about four-fifths (80 percent) of my plate is usually filled with alkaline-friendly foods and the other one-fifth (20 percent) of my plate has acidic foods. For example, four-fifths could be vegetables, legumes, and grains, while the rest of my plate might have bread or cheese.

All that said, do I expect you to switch to this type of diet full time? I'd love it if you did because I believe a plant-based diet is so important. Plus, a lot of alkaline foods in general are healthy for you, while many acid-forming foods tend not to be. I mean, whether you believe in the diet's theory or not, it's hard to deny that broccoli is better than candy for you, right? Believe me when I tell you that trying this is a great way to soothe your body from the inside out.

If you want to dip your toe into it for a day, start fifty-fifty (meaning, fill your plate with half alkaline foods and half acidic foods. Each time you try it, try your best to shift that ratio more toward the alkaline and away from the acidic. If you're not sure which group your favorite foods fall into, here's a quick list to start you off:

Alkaline foods

- **High alkalinity:** Alkaline water, barley grass, broccoli, broccoli sprouts, cucumbers, jicama, kale, kelp, parsley, radishes, soy sprouts, spinach, Himalayan salt.
- **Middle-of-the-road alkalinity:** Artichokes, arugula, asparagus, avocados, bee pollen, cauliflower, celery, cherries (sour), collard greens, flaxseed oil, garlic, green beans, green cabbage, lemons, lettuce, limes, mustard greens, parsnips, pumpkin, quinoa, squash, tomatoes, turnips, white cabbage.
- **Low alkalinity:** Almonds, beans (navy/white), beets, bell peppers, bok choy, bottled water, brussels sprouts, buckwheat pasta, carrots, coconut, edamame, grapefruit, lentils, olive oil, onions, organic tofu, peas, raw honey, red cabbage, yams, zucchini.

Acidic foods

- **High acidity:** Alcohol, artificial sweeteners, beef, candy, canned fruit, chocolate, coffee, dried fruits, eggs, fried foods, high-sodium foods, jelly and jam, pork, processed foods, shellfish, sweetened fruit juices, tuna, veal, vinegar.
- **Middle-of-the-road acidity:** Apples, apricots, bananas, blackberries, blueberries, brown rice, buffalo meat, butter,

cashews, chicken, cranberries, dry dates, dry figs, grapes, guava, ketchup, mangoes, mayonnaise, nectarines, oats, oranges, papyrus, peaches, pears, pineapples, pink grapefruit, raspberries, soda, strawberries, sweet cherries, whole-grain pasta, wild rice, yogurt (sweetened).
- **Low to neutral acidity:** Black beans, cantaloupe, chickpeas, cooked vegetables, green tea, hummus, oatmeal, sesame seeds, soybeans, sunflower seeds, watermelon, yogurt (unsweetened).

Soothe by curbing your nighttime nibbles. Because your body does a lot of its healing when you sleep, being smart about what types of foods you eat (and how much you eat in general) before you go to bed is so important. Choose wisely, and what's in your belly won't affect your forty winks, but making poorer choices can be disruptive and affect how long or how well you sleep. But there are better decisions you can make before bedtime to improve your odds of waking up feeling refreshed, recovered, and ready to take on your day.

- **Avoid eating too much:** Odds are anything above 200 calories eaten right before bedtime will only be stored as unwanted body fat. If you need to eat something, keep it around 100 to 150 calories.
- **Stay away from anything fatty or sweet:** Eating any foods with unhealthy (saturated) fats or added sugars could make you feel more alert, preventing you from falling asleep as easily.
- **Step away from anything reactionary:** Spicy or acidic foods (such as citrus or citrus juice) may not bother you when you eat or drink them, but they could disrupt your sleep by causing heartburn or other issues that could leave you feeling more tired in the morning as a result.
- **Stick with the right mix:** To keep your blood sugar levels even, pick something (or a combination of foods) that's a mix of complex

carbohydrates and either healthy fats or protein. For example, a slice of whole-grain bread with one or two ounces of fresh chicken, a serving of cottage cheese and a few almonds, a serving of Greek yogurt with a teaspoon of chia seeds, or a small apple with a half tbsp. of peanut butter.

Soothe your stress and anxiety. Call them "calming foods" if you like, but certain vegetables, fruits, and other edibles contain nutrients that help reduce anxiety and lower stress levels altogether. What's inside them can improve how your body responds to stress by triggering the release of "feel-good" chemicals, regulating your emotions, and reducing your stress hormones (specifically cortisol).

Now, chances are you're probably incorporating a few of these into your diet already. Even if that's the case, to pull off this "soothe," try adding a few more of the following into your day whenever possible. The more you do, the mellower you might find yourself.

- **Vitamin C–rich fruits and vegetables:** Whether you like the traditional suspects such as berries[1] and citrus fruits (oranges, grapefruit, tangerines, lemons, and limes) or prefer some of the lesser-known varieties (tomatoes, kale, broccoli, and green or yellow peppers), each one is loaded with vitamin C, which fights stress by reducing your cortisol levels.
- **Magnesium-dense foods:** Dark chocolate, broccoli, bananas, pumpkin seeds, spinach, and avocados are all rich in this mineral, which helps lower inflammation and metabolize cortisol. **Bonus points** if you pick **spinach** (which is also high in folate, a nutrient that triggers the production of dopamine, a neurotransmitter that helps reduce depression and stabilizes your mood) and **avocados** (known for lowering blood pressure and being packed with stress-fighting B vitamins).
- **Oatmeal and bananas:** Both contain L-tryptophan, an amino

acid that boosts the release of serotonin (a neurotransmitter responsible for mood regulation that helps create a feeling of relaxation and well-being in most people).[2]

- **Seeds and nuts:** Both have ample amounts of stress-fighting omega-3 fatty acids, which are great for boosting serotonin and reducing the level of cortisol in your system. Walnuts, flax seeds, and chia seeds are just a few good options, but if you want even more antianxiety insurance, lean toward cashews and sunflower seeds, since they also contain L-tryptophan.
- **Fatty fish (and shellfish):** Just like seeds and nuts, fatty fish, such as salmon, tuna, and halibut—as well as oysters, crabs, and mussels—are all high in omega-3 fatty acids, particularly DHA (docosahexaenoic acid), which helps nourish the brain and lower blood pressure.

Soothe by fortifying your fiber. If every meal or snack you eat is plant-based (or made from fruit, vegetables, or whole grains), then you're probably taking in a little fiber in every bite—and that's good. Even though I'll get into the serious science about why fiber is so healthy for you later, one of its many benefits is how it helps with digestion and keeps things moving through your body as efficiently as possible.

That benefit alone makes things a little less stressful on your body, which is why I'm a big fan of trying to sneak in fiber as often as possible throughout the day—and it really doesn't take much at all. In fact, just a tablespoon of lentils, a quarter cup of sauerkraut, a half of a carrot, a tablespoon of lima beans, or even a single teaspoon of unsweetened cocoa powder each contains one gram of fiber. Depending on what you're eating, you could easily throw certain fiber-rich foods on top of (or into) whatever you're eating to give your meal or snack a little boost and your body a little break. Some of the best fiber-fortified players out there that you can mix and match include:

Food	Amount	Fiber (grams)	Food	Amount	Fiber (grams)
Acorn squash	1 cup	9	Mustard greens	1 cup	5
Adzuki beans	1 cup	17	Navy beans	1 cup	19
Air-popped popcorn	3 cups	4	Orange	1 medium-size	4
Almonds	1 oz.	4	Parsnip	1 cup	6
Apple	1 medium-size	4	Peach	1 medium-size	2
Arugula	1 cup	.4	Peanuts	1 oz.	2
Asian pear	1 fruit	4	Pear	1 medium-size	6
Asparagus	3 spears	1	Peas	1 cup	14–16
Avocado	½ fruit	9	Pepper (green or yellow)	1 medium-size	2
Banana	1 medium-sized	3	Pinto beans	1 cup	15
Black beans	1 cup	15	Pistachio nuts	1 oz.	3
Blackberries	1 cup	8	Prunes	dried ½ cup	6
Blueberries	1 cup	4	Radicchio	1 leaf	.1
Brazil nuts	1 oz.	2	Raspberries	1 cup	8
Broccoli	1 cup	5	Red cabbage	1 cup	4
Brown rice	1 cup	4	Red potato	1 medium-size	3
Brussels sprouts	1 cup	6	Rice bran	1 oz.	6
Bulgur	1 cup	8	Russet potato	1 medium-size	4
Cashews	1 oz.	1	Sesame seeds	¼ cup	4
Cauliflower	1 cup	5	Spaghetti squash	1 cup	2
Collard greens	1 cup	8	Spinach	1 cup	4
Cranberry beans	1 cup	16	Starfruit	1 medium-size	2.5

Crookneck squash	1 cup	3	Strawberries	1 cup	3
Currants (red or white)	1 cup	5	Sunflower seeds	¼ cup	3
Dried apricots	1 cup	9	Sweet potato	1 medium-size	4
Dried figs	½ cup	7	Sweet white corn	1 large ear	4
Edamame	1 cup	8	Swiss chard	1 cup	4
Elderberries	1 cup	10	Walnuts	1 oz.	2
Endive	1 cup	1.5	Watercress	10 sprigs	.1
Flaxseed	1 oz.	8	Wheat bran	1 oz.	12
Garbanzo beans	1 cup	12	White beans	1 cup	19
Gooseberries	1 cup	6	Whole-wheat spaghetti	1 cup	6
Green beans	1 cup	3	Wild rice	1 cup	3
Jicama	1 cup	6	Yams	1 cup	6
Kale	1 cup	3	Yellow beans	1 cup	18
Kidney beans	1 cup	16	Yellow squash	1 cup	1.2
Lentils	½ cup	8	Zucchini	1 cup	3
Lima beans	1 cup	14			

Soothe—Your Activities

Taking a break from being active is a welcome change, but if you're the type who feels you always need to throw it in fifth gear because you're eager to see results, it can be tough to embrace anything that feels less extreme. But believe me, sometimes you just have to chill because that's also a part of a healthy lifestyle. More importantly, your body really—I mean *REALLY*—needs you to, whether you recognize it or not.

Whether you spoil yourself with just one of these soothing techniques or strive to incorporate all of them eventually, I can promise that you won't be moving backward by giving yourself a break every once in a while. In fact, you'll not only reap more results, but make your body more impervious to pain and injuries, as well as simultaneously feel more at ease and energized. It's a win-win for your mind and your muscles!

Soothe by knowing your limitations. Exercise is one of the best ways to relieve stress for a number of reasons, including lowering your blood pressure and triggering the release of endorphins (chemicals produced by the brain that increase feelings of euphoria and reduce pain). But too much of a good thing can be a bad thing—and working out is no exception to that rule.

Training too long, too much, or too intensely can make the effects of fitness counterproductive by not giving your body enough time to rest, rebuild, and repair. It's called overtraining, and it's never a place you want to find yourself, because when you push your body too hard, it increases your chances of injuring yourself and suppresses your immune system.

To make matters worse, your body starts working against you in other ways, including elevating your blood pressure, causing chronic inflammation, and even boosting your levels of cortisol—a hormone responsible for tearing down muscle and storing excess body fat.

The thing is, overtraining isn't always easy to spot because when it comes to pushing your body *too much*—whether from resistance training, cardiovascular exercise, sports, or any physical activity— we're all different from each other. I know a few diehard athletes who can go six days a week and they feel fine, while others I know burn out if they try to push themselves more than three times a week. Fortunately, there's an easy way to figure out whether you're pushing yourself too hard:

Look for the obvious symptoms. For me, one of the warning signs is when I suddenly stop being excited about exercising and start doing things to avoid it. But if you hate exercise altogether, you probably never get excited about working out. So instead, pay attention to the following changes in yourself:

- Persistent fatigue
- A gradual (or sudden) drop in performance
- Constant moodiness (easily irritated)
- Feelings of depression or anxiety
- Sleep issues (insomnia or restlessness)
- Loss of appetite
- A suppressed immune system (meaning you notice an increase in getting colds, infections, or aches/pains)
- Lack of motivation or interest
- Muscle soreness that never goes away

Listen to your pulse. First, you need a baseline to start with. So, as soon as you wake up in the morning (and before you get yourself moving around), sit up in bed, take your pulse for sixty seconds, then write down that number. Continue doing that every morning and look for changes the morning after your workouts. If your pulse ever rises more than eight bpm (beats per minute) above your baseline, chances are you may need an extra day or two of rest, even if you're not experiencing any of the symptoms I mentioned earlier.

Soothe by being more flexible. Stretching is one of those activities that people really underestimate. You don't realize how much better you'll feel until you actually do it. For example, I'm not always aware when I'm walking around with tight hips or a tight lower back—I just know I'm not as comfortable throughout the day. But when I remember to stretch them, I instantly feel so much better! It's almost ridiculous how good it feels, but it's funny how stretching—even though I know I'll feel so much better afterward—is still something even I have to remind myself to do.

Stretching isn't just about loosening up your muscles to feel less tight and to reduce your risk of injury. It prevents postural issues that occur when certain muscles tighten up (specifically within your spine, knees, and shoulders) which can cause them to shift out of alignment. That's never a place you want your body to be, because your muscles are meant to work *with* (not against) each other. When they're out of alignment, your muscles are prevented from properly collectively absorbing force, which then shifts that force into your ligaments, discs, meniscus, bones, and joints. Over time, this leaves those areas weaker, inflamed (causing chronic pain), and more injury prone.

Stretching also helps alleviate stress by releasing feel-good endorphins, stimulating blood circulation, and even improving your balance, your coordination, and maybe best of all, your range of motion, which allows your muscles to recruit additional muscle fibers when you resistance train. (More fibers mean more overall development!)

So, what should you *do—and how should you do it?* There are basically four types of stretching: ballistic, proprioceptive neuro-muscular facilitation (PNF), dynamic, and static. The first three are pretty intense, have a higher risk of injury, and are generally recommended for intermediate to advanced exercisers and athletes. Your smartest and safest bet is static stretching, which is when you position your body in a certain way, then hold that pose for a specific amount of time.

Now, which stretches you pick is your choice, so long as you include at least one stretch for each of the following muscle groups: upper back, lower back, chest, shoulders, abdominals, hips, quadriceps, hamstrings, and calves. If you're not sure which to choose, I'm going to recommend a few you can start with. But whatever you pick, stick with the following rules:

1. Warm up your muscles for at least five minutes so they're more pliable. So, right after your resistance or cardio training, after a warm bath/shower, or just marching in place while pumping your arms back and forth.

2. Ease into each move and only stretch your muscles to the point of slight tightness or slight discomfort. You never want to force any movement to the point where you feel pain.

3. Once you're in position, hold the stretch for at least ten to thirty seconds. Personally, I always recommend holding a stretch for a little longer if you can (thirty seconds to a minute) because that's when you really start to feel tighter muscles release.

The Stretches

Perform each of these movements in any order you wish, doing each stretch at least once (up to three or four times).

1. Loosen up your chest (and shoulders) by . . .

Standing next to the edge of a wall with your left side closest to the wall, place your left hand flat against the wall, extending your left arm straight out, elbow unlocked. Step forward until you feel a slight stretch along the outside of your chest. Hold the stretch, then change positions and repeat the move with your right arm.

2. Loosen up your lower back (and spine) by . . .

Lying flat on your back with legs extended, bend your left knee and place your left foot flat on the floor. Grab the outside of your left knee with your right hand, then extend your left arm out to the side, placing your palm flat on the floor for support.

Keeping your left leg bent, gently pull your left knee over to your right as you simultaneously twist your torso to the left. Hold the stretch, slowly twist yourself back, then switch positions to repeat the stretch. Bend your right knee and grab it with your left hand, then gently pull your right knee to the left as you twist your torso to the right.

3. Loosen up your upper back by . . .

Putting your hands together by lacing your fingers together, then straighten your arms in front of you—as you do, gently rotate your hands so that your palms face away from you. Keeping your arms extended, gently tuck your chin down toward your chest and hold the stretch.

4. Loosen up your shoulders (and upper back) by . . .

Facing a wall that's far enough away from you so you can only touch it with your fingertips, slowly crawl your fingers up the wall like a spider, moving closer to the wall as you go, until your arms are raised as high as they can go. Hold the stretch, then slowly reverse the movement until you're back in the starting position.

5. Loosen up your quadriceps by . . .

Sitting on your heels, bring your arms behind you and put your palms on the floor—fingertips pointing away—a few inches behind your feet. Keeping your palms on the floor, gently tilt your pelvis up, then slowly lift your hips and chest as high as you can. (You'll also feel the movement in your back, shoulders, neck, and abdominals.) Hold the stretch, then slowly lower yourself back down.

6. Loosen up your hamstrings by . . .

Sitting on the floor with your legs extended in front of you, bend at the waist and reach forward as far as you comfortably can toward your feet—then hold the stretch.

Next, keeping your right leg straight, bend your left leg and place the sole of your left foot flat against the inside of your right thigh. Once again, bend at the waist and reach forward as far as you can, this time toward your right foot. Hold the stretch, then switch positions to repeat, this time keeping your left leg extended while placing the sole of your right foot against the inside of your left thigh.

7. Loosen up your hips by . . .

Getting on all fours with your knees together and palms on the floor, slightly wider than shoulder-width apart. Without raising your hands or knees, slowly rock your hips from side to side. As you go, imagine you're trying to lower your hips as close to the ground as possible.

NOTE: This stretch is harder to hold for long periods of time, so just concentrate on moving as slowly as possible, pausing for a few seconds each time you shift from side to side.

8. Loosen up your calves by . . .

Standing with your feet shoulder-width apart, step forward with your left foot. Place your hands on top of your left leg (just above your knee), then slowly straighten your right leg until your right heel is flat to the floor. As you hold the stretch, concentrate on keeping your back straight and your head up. Afterward, switch positions (right leg forward, left leg behind you) and repeat.

9. Loosen up your abdominals (and spine) by . . .

Lying flat on your stomach with your legs straight and the tops of your feet flat on the floor, bend your arms and place your palms flat on the floor just outside your shoulders. Keeping your hips and legs on the floor, slowly straighten your arms and press yourself up, raising your chin and looking up as you go as far as you comfortably can. Hold the stretch, then lower yourself back down.

Soothe your mind with meditation. There are many forms of meditation. In fact, even being an athlete is sort of a type of meditation for me. When I'm practicing on the court, I'm repeating the same thing over and over and over again. And as I do that, I start to go into what I call a "flow state," where I escape my thoughts by focusing on what my body's doing in that moment—and it feels great.

I know for some of you, meditation might seem too passive to be effective, but I'm not recommending it because of how it alleviates stress, lowers blood pressure, improves sleep quality, and even makes your immune system more efficient (among so many other benefits I'll get into in a later chapter). It's about slowing your life down—even if it's just for a few minutes—because you deserve it.

So, what should *you* do—and how should you do it? There are so many different methods for relaxing the mind—from guided, mantra, and transcendental meditation to more physical forms, such as tai chi or qigong—that it's really your choice what works for you, in my opinion. A fast and easy version of meditation that anyone can do without much effort is a form of mindfulness meditation, where your main goal is essentially to just focus on the now.

Before you try this, just remember not to think about the process too much. I mean, overthinking about whether you're doing it right defeats the purpose of trying to relax your mind in the first place. So, try the following tips, but don't panic if you can't pull them off perfectly. The more you practice meditation, the less you'll worry about doing it perfectly and, ironically, you'll end up doing it more effectively without really needing to think too hard about it.

- *Wear clothing as relaxed as you hope to be.* Meaning, if you're new to meditation, change into clothes that aren't restricting in any way. Even though you won't be moving, you don't want anything on your body that might distract you.
- *Find a distraction-free spot.* This one might be easier said than done, but find a place where you won't be bothered by anyone and that's preferably as quiet as possible.
- *Do it at the best time possible*. If that's first thing in the morning, as soon as you get home from work, or just before bedtime, it really doesn't matter. But to get more bang for your buck, choose a time when your mind really could benefit from slowing down.
- *Carve out enough time.* Even ten minutes of meditation can make a big difference, so dedicate at least that much to start and don't shoot for more until you're ready.
- *Position yourself anyway you want.* You don't have to sit cross-legged with your hands on your lap if that's not comfortable for you. Instead, get in whatever seated position works best for your

body. (And if you need back support, use a chair, or sit on the floor and lean against the wall.)

- *Finally, focus on your breathing.* But don't overdo it. What I mean by that is just breathe as slowly as possible through your nose and exhale from your mouth. As you go, don't worry if you're going too fast or about doing anything wrong. Just be aware of your breathing, feel your lungs expanding and contracting with each breath, and if any thoughts pop into your head, acknowledge them, then let them float away without dwelling on them.

As a final point, don't go into this expecting instant results immediately afterward. If you meditate as I'm suggesting, it will naturally reduce levels of adrenaline and cortisol in your system throughout the entire process—that's a given. But you should feel calmer and less anxious—a little more centered and a lot less scattered—than when you started.

Soothe—Who and What's Around You

Your friends, your family, the people who orbit your world may have an impact on you, but you also have an impact on them. And just as you can enrich their lives, you also have the power to soothe the relationship you have with them. No matter how close we might be to someone, no matter how deep those roots may run, we all hit a snag with someone now and then. But you can control whether tempers flare or feathers go up—all it takes are the right words, approach, and attitude.

Soothe by sitting on your reactions. When you think about it, how many fights have you ever had with anyone that you didn't laugh about later with that person? If you're like most people, you've probably blown up and made up with someone more times than you've blown up and never spoken to someone again.

If that's you, then acknowledge it, but think about this: When it comes to most of those kiss and make up arguments, whatever it was you were fighting about probably wasn't terrible enough to take down the relationship. If you came to a compromise afterward, it just took a little time to get there—so why not make an effort to shrink down that time?

Whenever a conflict arises, the first thing most of us focus on is how that situation makes us feel, but that causes you to lead with an emotional reaction instead of a realistic one. In other words, we start thinking with our hearts instead of our heads. That's when the words that come out of our mouths might not be what we'd say if calmer heads prevailed—and things just start snowballing out of control from there.

See, I'm one of those people, who, for the most part, knows what they want to say, especially if I'm close to someone. But at some point, I realized that whenever I would have disagreements with longtime friends, my sister, parents, and partners—those were times when I *really* needed to hold things in and think about them first. I'm not saying to hold things in for too long, because that's when it starts to become toxic. I just think about them for enough time to thoroughly shape my opinion and minimize any unnecessary conflicts. I also found out through trial and error that you can't avoid conflict—you must confirm what the opposing message is, then be honest about needing more time to process that message, even if you don't necessarily side with their opinion.

Instead of reacting to how another person is making you *feel* during an argument, take a pause, hold your tongue, and literally let them talk themselves out. (I don't care how much time it takes, but they will eventually run out of things to say.) As they speak, forget about their tone, and try to look for the message they're trying to send between all the words they may not mean, then, if possible, tell them you'd like some time to reflect on what they've said. However, if the situation doesn't allow you to take time to sleep on it, try repeating back what the person said by saying something such as, "Let me see if I understand you correctly. What you feel is [insert what they said here], do I have that right?" Just that simple act can defuse the situation by proving that you're actively listening to their words and genuinely acknowledging what's concerning them.

It takes practice—and trust me, it takes patience—but making these conscious efforts will not only keep things from escalating but it will leave the other person feeling heard, even if you don't agree with what they have to say.

Soothe by changing someone's mood. Hey, we all have days we're on top and plenty of other days when we feel like we're at rock bottom. If that's happening to you, then guess what? It's happening to everyone else too, including the people you care about. And if someone you care about is walking around all bleak and gloom-ridden, then they're not doing anyone else any favors—especially you. Negative energy feeds negative energy, so try to nip that in the bud.

Whenever you see someone who's typically cheery and hopeful but currently down in the dumps, make a conscious effort to bring them back to that place. Often, just being straight with them about what they're projecting, then asking what you can do works wonders. Seriously, if they're close to your heart, you should be able to say, "Hey, listen, I know you're feeling down, but you're bringing others down too—and I know you don't mean to do that. So, is there any way I can help you so that you're not in that position?"

Sometimes doing that can pop them out of their attitude simply because you're making them aware of what they're presenting or because you're showing them support. Other times, they may genuinely need someone in that moment, and once you step in to help, you can make it easier for them to flip that switch back over from negative to positive.

Soothe by being happy with zero. Like I said in the "Balance" chapter of the book, the people you bring into your circle are the relationships that need to be mutually beneficial for both of you. But you can't always expect that things are going to be even stephen all the time. It's a common myth that a healthy relationship should always be fifty-fifty, but sometimes one person will carry the burden more than the other for a certain period.

There will be days when you're not immediately thanked for doing something nice for someone. There will be times when you're not acknowledged whatsoever for being courteous and considerate. And, there will be moments when you put forth more effort than the person you consider your friend. As long as the two of you remain dedicated to each other, it can still be a fruitful relationship. Just remember that so long as it's not a consistent reaction to your kindness, then it's just a day, it's just a time, and it's just a moment—nothing more.

Sure, in a perfect world, we would all appreciate every single act of support and compassion shown to us by stopping and thanking every single person responsible, but that's a perfect world. It's just natural that sometimes when you're generous and encouraging to others, they might not recognize what you're doing in that moment. But instead of obsessing about why they didn't appreciate you, remind yourself that it was never about being acknowledged—you did what you did because you cared about that person.

You see, by becoming preoccupied with why somebody didn't thank you, it can sometimes keep you from wanting to repeat similar acts of kindness not just toward them but toward others. Before you know it, that negative energy can start working its way into other relationships, all because you weren't admired in that tiny moment.

Instead, don't expect a trophy to be handed to you the next time you do something kind for a friend, and remind yourself to be happy with zero. If those zeroes start adding up, then sure, you might need to reconsider the relationship. But if they don't, accept it for what it is and power through, but continue to always say thank you to that person in the future. Not just because it's the right thing to do but because of how it may inspire others who see you do it—or even change the behavior of that specific person later on.

Soothe by sharing more of yourself. Whether we realize it or not, most people tend to open up more to those who open up more to them. At times, it's healthy to drop your guard, allow yourself to be vulnerable, and share something personal with people around you. It doesn't have to be anything controversial or tabloid worthy. Just something that reminds them that you trust them with who you really are.

Some people have what I would call *share-itis* because they overshare, but I'm the exact opposite. I think you have to pick and choose when to share by reading the room first, because if the room is feeling like ice, then there won't be any sharing. (LOL!) But when it's not and the moment's right, you could end up helping someone else and/or build a deeper and stronger friendship by doing so.

For example, I have this friend and we were hanging tough, hanging heavy, and hitting balls all the time. But I went through a three-day period when I didn't have time to call him, and it strangely changed the friendship. We didn't talk about what happened for a year and a half because he was upset with me, but I finally asked him to sit down with me at a restaurant and talk about it. I told him, "Look, this is a superficial friendship if we can't even figure out what's going on with one another. If we're going to be friends, we really need to tell each other what's honestly happening in our lives."

So we did, and trust me, we could have shared even more but it had gotten so late, we had the waiters giving us the evil eye to go home. But it felt so nice to finally have that long overdue conversation because it helped me a lot. You have to keep growing as a person—and that means emotionally too.

Soothe—Yourself

When you're always on the go, it can be hard to take a few minutes to slow down. Maybe it's because it can sometimes feel selfish or lazy to steal a little "me time." Other days, you may not have any time to even stop for a second—or at least you think you don't. Whatever the excuse, you have to remind yourself of the importance of putting your life on pause once in a while to focus on what heals you mentally, spiritually, and physically.

It's also part of the secret sauce that helps relieve stress, reduce inflammation, and lessen any aches and pains. But most importantly, it's about taking that moment because you deserve that moment—and don't you forget that.

Soothe by carving out a "just say no" night. At least once a week, no matter how busy I am, I do what I like to call a "just say no" night. It might be saying no to a party, an event, a dinner— something that might be fun to do, and it's not like I don't love the people who will be there, but I take that break to keep myself on track.

I consider it sort of preventative medicine because, before I brought this into my life, I was always triple booked and going out every single night. So many times, I'd wait until I was seriously run-down to the point where I'd get sick before finally having the strength to give myself a night off. But by then, everything was off, including my eating habits, my energy, my sleep, and especially my health.

But when you play that sort of "get out of jail free" card on a regular basis—when you give one night a week just to yourself, no matter how tempting it is to go out or who asks you—you'll be surprised at how allowing yourself to just chill once a week magically keeps everything in place.

Soothe by breathing every hour. Sure, you're breathing all the time because you have to—some say around seventeen thousand times a day—but do you even realize what your body is doing with all that air? Every single cell in your body requires oxygen—that's right, I said every cell—so the more oxygen you're able to take in, the more benefit you bring to literally every single part of yourself. It's crazy to think about, but once you realize that every time you inhale and exhale, you're in complete control of something that affects your entire body—doesn't it make more sense to give it more than you usually do?

Look, I'm not expecting you to get more by breathing as deeply as possible every single time—I mean, we are talking seventeen thousand here! Ideally, I want you to always turn to this technique: Focus on taking six or seven deep breaths every hour—slowly drawing in as much air as possible through your nose, holding it for a second or two, then slowly exhaling from your mouth. This small exercise will go a long way toward making you feel more energized than you felt prior to showing some love to your airflow.

Soothe by taking a nap if possible. I love naps—well, who doesn't. In fact, whenever I'm traveling, it's crucial for me to get one in right after I land to adjust to jet lag and any performance issues that could occur because of it. But there's a lot more to naps than just reducing fatigue and restoring alertness. When you can do it, it's an incredible recovery tool that simultaneously helps rejuvenate and heal your body.

The science is out there on how a nap not only helps to reduce stress but can significantly reduce sleep deprivation, which by itself can impair memory, elevate cortisol levels, and even slow down your metabolism. But making the most of a nap isn't as easy as just putting your head down. The length of a nap is just as important as when you take it, because if you get it wrong, you can just as easily experience the opposite effect. Here is the best course of action:

- **Keep an eye on the clock.** The sweet spot in terms of timing is thought to be when your body temperature typically drops during the day—around midafternoon between 1 p.m. to 3 p.m.
- **Keep it short—around ten to thirty minutes max.** If you go any longer, you increase your chances of falling into a deeper sleep, which could disrupt your nighttime sleeping or leave you feeling more exhausted after your nap instead of refreshed.

Soothe by being a friend to yourself. I'm just going to come right out and say it. Somewhere along this journey, maybe the first month, week, or even first day—you're going to screw it up. And even though I told you to appreciate every loss, this lesson is about learning from your mistakes—it's about cutting yourself some slack for making them.

How would you react to a good friend who screwed up but didn't mean to? What would you say to someone close to you who struggled to pull off what they had hoped to accomplish? Would you beat them up for it? Make them feel terrible about themselves for failing? Shake your head when they tried their best? Of course you wouldn't—so come on, why does it make any sense to do it to yourself?

Don't get me wrong, I want you to push yourself as hard as you can. But if you can't do what you set out to do on certain days, don't belittle yourself, but be your best friend instead. Pick yourself up just as you would a friend who fell. Treat yourself exactly as you would treat someone else by being kind to yourself and appreciating what you've accomplished, no matter how little that might be on that day.

CHAPTER 8

BELIEVE

I'm always flattered when people comment that I have a distinct, unmistakable style. Something unique that shows in my game, my sense of fashion, my interior design work—the way I carry myself and live my life. But what may seem "distinct" or "unique" to others isn't something I've ever thought hard about or paid much attention to. All I've ever done is embrace who I was and remain confident in the direction I was moving in my life.

In other words, all I ever do is **believe** in the actions and behaviors that make me who I am and help move me forward, which is something within everyone's reach. Because we all have a "distinct, unmistakable style." It's just that so few of us ever believe in ourselves or the actions we're taking to try and improve our lives enough to allow it to shine through.

That lack of faith is what causes so many to fail with their health and wellness goals—even if the game plan they're following is a good one. They don't understand how the simple act of believing in themself and also believing in the process that they've put in place helps exponentially when it comes to every aspect of their life, whether it's maintaining a healthier diet, developing better personal habits, being more active, and so on.

That's what this action is all about—getting you to trust yourself and the steps you're taking each day. Some of the actions I want you to tackle in this section might seem trivial, and because of that, you may be tempted to skip them, but don't make that mistake. This is one of the eight actions behind STRIVE for a reason. It will remind you to remain confident that the healthier decisions you're making now are going to pay off later. Maybe not today. Maybe not tomorrow. But eventually, depending on you and your conviction, the returns around the corner are absolutely worth the investment.

This section is also about the powerful relationship that your mind has with your body. If you're not spiritual and don't hold much stock in the whole "mind-body connection," I get that. But even if that's not your thing, there's no denying that your brain is the control center for everything. And because of that, whether we like it or not, how we feel and the way we think directly affects our health and physical well-being. The more you believe in the process, the more it will work for you instead of against you.

Believe—The Right Way

The fact is I'm asking you to believe that if you follow these eight actions, your life will change significantly for the better. But let's be real here. It's one thing to tell someone to believe in the steps needed to improve themselves—and an entirely different animal to get them to. For some people, getting to that "place of belief" isn't just challenging but the hardest tenet of the eight because it requires a lot of optimism that you might not have. If that's you, and don't worry if it is because you're not alone, I want you to consider the following as you move through this section:

Don't be scared—be excited. When we really want something—when we want real change—it can be intimidating, right? We're often not sure how we're going to get where we want to go because, to get there, it typically means traveling a road we've never taken before—or one we've been on once before but got lost. Even as you begin making positive changes in your life, you may start questioning yourself: "Can I really change the way I think? The way I eat? The things I do? The time I have? Can I actually feel confident about myself and what I'm doing?"

The answer is yes. You can because, once you start to STRIVE, no matter what options you choose to try and what direction you decide to take, you're going to begin building habits by reinforcing certain actions repeatedly—just like an athlete.

That's basically all an athlete does. No one ever starts perfect—and no one starts being the best at something immediately. All any athlete ever does is get out there and do something over and over and over again. They start by being average. And then good. And, if they put enough time in and believe in themselves and the steps they're taking, then they end up great. That's going to be you, so long as you believe in the process.

If you've failed before—forget about that. Part of what keeps some people from believing in the process is remembering other moments in their life when they didn't succeed. When they might have tried to change their life for the better—and wholeheartedly believed in the process—but ultimately, things didn't turn out as expected. But if you keep thinking about past failures, those failures will prevent you from having the faith to try once again to move forward.

Whether you choose to let yourself recognize it or not, you *do* have the strength within yourself to change what you're presently doing for the better. It's not that you're special—it's simply because everybody has that ability. Anybody can decide if they're going to make good or bad choices on any given day.

And guess what? Everybody also has a history of failure with something. So, you're not alone, but the difference between winners and losers is that winners learn from failure and then let it fade away. As you STRIVE, you will fail at certain moments, but I want you to learn from each failure—and then don't give it a second thought.

If you lose faith—remember the facts. Even when we know what's good for us, it can be easy to talk ourselves out of doing it. We can make ourselves believe that "trying this" or "changing that" might make a huge difference in others' lives but really won't have an impact in our lives because, well, our circumstances are different from everybody else's.

That's why this section is heavily loaded with some of the science that supports many of the changes that I'm suggesting you try. So, in moments when you have a harder time finding and tapping into that confidence that exists within you, dig deeper into this portion of the book to find more reassurance in the research.

Believe—In Your Diet

So, confession time—I was a yo-yo dieter. Although I hate to admit it, there have been so many moments throughout my life when I would fall off the "health train" and eat junk food for weeks on end. I never really went past a month of eating that way, but whenever I fell off, even though it was just for a short period, I never quite bounced back the same. By that time, the damage was already done in regard to how I felt and how I looked.

What helped me conquer my yo-yo eating was finally understanding that I'm *going* to fall off the rails eventually. It's inevitable and there's absolutely no shame in that. The only crime was *staying off* the train. Because if you wait too long to try to get back on, that train will be gone and all the way in California—and you're still stuck in Missouri!

A great example is when I went to Disney World with my family a couple years ago. Sugar is such a trigger for me. I can't be around it. I can't keep it in my home, because if it's there, I'm going to eat it, and when I do, I'm not pacing myself.

The first day we were there, I was good and just had popcorn. The next day, I let myself have *one* sugar-based treat. But that third day, we went to Epcot. I had never been there before, and at first I was like, "Let's just *try* something sweet," as a treat for the event. I would take a bite and let it go. But a couple hours later, I literally left my family to go eat junk food.

I was just walking around Epcot buying, tasting, and eating pretty much everything I could. I even called a friend to tell him about a Lucky Charms milkshake I found to ask him if I should try it because it was his favorite, and he said, "Yeah, go for it!" It was a disaster because I couldn't even eat dinner with my family later on. But on that day, I decided to just let go and accept it knowing that the very next day, I would get right back to where I was before that downward spiral.

Now when I fall off, I give myself *that* day—no self-shaming or guilt allowed—but I get back on the very next day instead of letting things spiral out of control for weeks. To help me believe in the process and jump on the train faster, I'll go back and refresh my memory about why certain key nutrients are so important for me, and how what I'm eating now really does makes a difference, even if I can't see those behind-the-scenes benefits immediately.

Believe that fiber has your back. Right now, nine out of ten Americans aren't getting enough fiber. The reason is because the traditional Western diet isn't very fiber rich, which is tragic because the long-term health benefits of getting enough fiber in your diet are hard to ignore.

What makes it magical is that it's a carbohydrate your body can't break down and comes in two forms: soluble (which dissolves in water and is found in vegetables, beans, nuts and seeds, oats, barley, and certain fruits such as apples and strawberries) and insoluble (which stays intact in water and is found in vegetables, beans, whole grains, brown rice, bulgur, wheat bran, nuts, and many vegetables). Both forms sweep through your digestive system and move things along.

I believe that's one reason some people dismiss fiber. Too many people associate the nutrient as being the one you turn to if you're concerned about your bowel movements or because it leaves you feeling fuller (and less inclined to overeat or snack). Sure, they're not wrong, but if you don't feel you have a problem with staying regular or overeating, then you might feel you don't really need to monitor how much fiber you're getting during the day.

But fiber is your friend for so many reasons beyond satiety. It absorbs excess calories (so your body stores less fat), lowers blood pressure and LDL in your system (the "bad" type of cholesterol), and keeps your blood sugar levels stable. It's also a major player in reducing your risk of a variety of conditions, including diabetes, cardiovascular inflammation, heart disease, and even certain cancers. It's why I consider it a true head-to-toe body soother.

Whenever I feel I need a little reminder in believing in the importance of fiber, all it takes is reminding myself that the World Health Organization proved that, for every eight grams of dietary fiber, the total number of deaths and frequency of type 2 diabetes, coronary heart disease, and colorectal cancer drops between 5 to 27 percent.[1] All of that from just eight grams! That's literally eating just an orange and one ounce of almonds, or an apple and two ounces of peanuts. No excuses!

Believe in the power of fat. For some people, being asked to have some type of healthy fat in every meal or snack feels a little off, especially if one of their goals is to lose weight. And sure, while it's true that one gram of fat contains nine calories (protein and carbohydrates are only four calories per gram), doubting the process and shying away from fat because you're afraid it will make you heavier or unhealthy is the wrong attitude to take.

Granted, not all types of fat are necessarily good for you. The bad kinds are trans fats (typically abundant in animal products, fast foods, or any food that contains hydrogenated oils) and saturated fats (the kind you'll find in dairy, beef, pork, lamb, butter, poultry with skin, eggs, and vegetable fats that remain liquid at room temperature, such as coconut and palm oil). I'm not saying to completely remove these from your diet. I'm just saying that the less of it you eat, the better.

But the good kinds—unsaturated fats—well, they're a different story. Unsaturated fats come in two types: monounsaturated fats (MUFAs) and polyunsaturated fats (PUFAs). Both are good for you when eaten in moderation, playing a major role in keeping your body temperature regulated, reducing inflammation, protecting your organs, maintaining healthy skin and hair, helping your body absorb certain key vitamins (particularly A, D, E, and K), and repairing and protecting the walls around every cell within your body. In other words, the "good" fats are your friends, so don't fear them.

Believe in healing through hydration. Staying hydrated sort of suffers from being attached to weight loss in the same way fiber does. Yes, drinking plenty of water all day long can leave you feeling fuller and keep you from reaching for food (and calories) you don't necessarily need, but the advantages beyond that obvious perk are seriously astronomical.

Literally every system in your entire body requires water to operate properly—every system! When you hydrate, all that water goes to work to help transport vitamins, minerals, and other nutrients to your cells, flush out harmful toxins, steady your blood pressure, and regulate your body temperature, on top of cushioning your organs and joints against shock and injuries.

It's so crucial that letting yourself lose as little as just 1 percent of your body weight in water can disrupt your body's metabolism (so you burn fewer calories all day long) and prevent you from delivering as much oxygen throughout your body (which can lead to fatigue that impacts your all-day activity). One percent! Think about that for a moment. If you weigh 150 pounds, that's just twenty-four ounces (the same amount of liquid as two cans of soda). You could easily and quickly lose that amount on a hot day or just going to the bathroom, and it's a loss that can cause a decrease in your overall performance between 10 to 20 percent.

That's why every time you take a sip, I want you to try and think about hydration's impact on your body. You need to believe that staying well hydrated not only means you're keeping every function within your body operating efficiently, but that you're giving yourself more energy. Energy that will help you bring even more effort to exercise and whatever activities you choose to keep yourself in shape with later.

Believe in those fruits and veggies. Did you know research shows that people who eat three vegetables a day live on average around two and a half years longer than those that don't eat vegetables?[2] Or that for every fifty cents you spend on fruits and vegetables, your risk of all-cause mortality could drop between 10 to 12 percent?[3] If you did, it was still worth mentioning. And if you didn't, well, that's the point.

I don't have to tell you that fresh fruits and vegetables are an abundant source of vitamins, minerals, antioxidants, fiber, enzymes, and other equally health-friendly nutrients. Could I hit you with research paper after research paper about how having them in your diet has been proven to lower your risk of countless types of cancer, heart disease and stroke, and a variety of other life-threatening chronic diseases? Yeah, I guess, but I'm not here to play the mom card on you. Besides, you probably know these things because they've been drilled into you all your life—but are you really drinking it in?

Look, I'm not expecting you to be an expert on every fruit and vegetable to help you truly believe in why they're so special. I get it. That's a lot to absorb, especially because there are literally thousands of different fruits and vegetables out there, each with its own unique mix of nutrients and at least a few hundred studies explaining how important that particular fruit or vegetable is for your health. Studies that go back decades—studies that are being performed right now as you read this. So, what are you waiting for? Use all that knowledge to deepen your beliefs.

What I mean is this: Instead of just blindly eating vegetables and fruits each day because you've been told to, try reminding yourself *in the moment* how your body is about to profit from that food right before you eat it. I mean it—grab your phone, type the name of the food in, along with the words *health benefits*, then really absorb what pops up when you search. (So long as the information is from a reputable source, such as the USDA National Nutrient Database, the US Food and Drug Administration, the American Cancer Society, the American Heart Association, or the Mayo Clinic, just to name a few.)

When you do this every time—and I mean every time—it helps to kind of "wake you up" to why you're doing this. It's an instant way to restore your faith in the foods you're choosing. And it's crazy, but it can honestly make you more eager to eat that food than you felt seconds before—it can even make that fruit or vegetable taste better—and that's what I want for you. I want you reaching for these foods not because you're told to but because you know about and believe in the benefits they're bringing to your body.

Believe—In Your Activities

'm the type who couldn't imagine not being active, but maybe that's not you—and that's fair. For a lot of people, having to exercise regularly isn't much fun at all, even if the benefits far outweigh the boredom. It might be why over 73 percent of all adults over twenty in the United States are overweight, with close to 42 percent of that total considered obese (according to the Centers for Disease Control and Prevention).[4] But reminding yourself often about what's happening to your body because of all the effort you're putting into it can make believing in the importance of staying active a little easier.

Believe you can reverse your age. Whether you like it or not, the facts are the facts. As soon as you celebrate your thirtieth birthday, science shows your body begins losing muscle—as much as 3 to 5 percent every decade (about a half pound a year on average). That gradual loss isn't just making you weaker but it also slows down your metabolism—so you burn fewer calories at rest and store the rest as unwanted body fat. Not a good trade off. But when you balance your resistance training by doing it two to three times a week, you can prevent that muscle loss and even boost your metabolism by as much as 15 percent.

Now look, I have friends who are just naturally thin and couldn't care less about having lean muscle. And if that's you, I'll tell you the same thing I say to them: Yes, resistance training helps make your muscles grow, but it also reverses aging by stabilizing your joints and improving your mobility and balance. The same load-bearing exercises that build muscle also work to support bone density, making them incredibly effective at reducing your risk of osteoporosis. In fact, resistance training doesn't just help prevent the bone loss that occurs naturally as we age—it may even help build new bone! Beyond all that, it's also been shown to reduce your chances of developing heart disease and diabetes, as well as to lower levels of LDL cholesterol, the bad kind that clogs your arteries. In other words, the same program that is helping you build lean muscle you might not care about is making your entire body healthier at the same time.

Believe that you can keep your heart healthy. I mentioned earlier in this book that 150 minutes a week of cardiovascular activity is what the Centers for Disease Control and Prevention recommends, right? Well, if you need even more evidence why you need to believe in that number, know that research has already proven that doing any form of exercise—and I mean any kind of exercise—at least 150 minutes a week could add as much as five years to your life.[5]

How can that be possible? Well, according to the Mayo Clinic,[6] being consistent with your cardio prevents you from being overweight, conditions your heart, reduces your blood pressure, increases high-density lipoprotein (HDL) cholesterol (the "good" kind) in your system, and keeps your cholesterol in check, among plenty of other life-extending benefits. In fact, all those positives may explain why regular exercise has been proven to lower your risk of certain types of cancer (such as breast and colon cancer), hypertension, strokes, diabetes, and many other chronic diseases and medical conditions.

If the stuff you can't see yet is hard to believe in, then believe in the stuff you can spot right away. Not only will you see a noticeable difference in your all-day energy but regular cardiovascular training also improves the quality of your sleep and helps flush away lactic acid, the leftover toxins resistance training creates that cause that burning sensation you sometimes feel during and after you train. Every time you feel like you have more steam, enjoy a better night's sleep, or seem a little less sore, let those obvious rewards serve as little reminders that you can believe how hard cardio's working secretly inside you to improve your overall health.

Believe in the benefits of sitting and chilling. If meditation feels too easy to be effective, you need to change that mindset right now. We're so conditioned to think that, in order to see results, we need to put in a lot of work. And just lying there, breathing in and out, doesn't seem that hard to do.

But let me stop you right there—is it really that easy? Because most people I know can't seem to carve out any time for themselves to meditate. We're all too obsessed with getting things done that we don't have any time to literally do "nothing," if that's all that you think meditation is. For most of us, it's not easy because we never give ourselves that time.

But when you do, regular meditation has been proven to impact both your body and your brain in ways you may not even realize. Yeah, you already know that it helps reduce depression, anxiety, and stress. And forget about how it lowers resting heart rate and blood pressure (including your diastolic[7] and systolic[8] blood pressure), or its power to help you sleep better and even reduce your risk of suffering from insomnia.[9] I'm talking about the added bonuses that taking a breath every once in a while can bring.

Because of meditation's ability to lower chronic psychological stress, that impact could improve your immune cells and boost your immune system according to research.[10] Plus, not only does it calm your mind, but it also boosts your brain's cognitive function,[11] blood flow,[12] and the production of myelin[13]—a protective layer of fats that cover nerve cells. On top of all that, meditation has been proven to lower inflammation,[14] reduce emotional eating urges,[15] and make it easier to manage chronic pain.[16] All that and so much more, just by stepping away from the chaos for a little while on a regular basis.

Believe in how steps move you forward. First, remember this fact if you don't believe in the power of walking. Just because you might be moving at a slower pace doesn't mean you're not using the same muscles when you walk that you rely on when running (your quadriceps, hamstrings, glutes, calves, and core). Plus, your body burns roughly one hundred calories per mile whether you run that distance or walk it. I don't know about you, but I know which choice I would prefer, especially when you realize the impact of every step (and the shock to your joints) when you run is six times greater than walking.

Even though it's not as brutal on your body as jogging or running, that doesn't mean it doesn't bring the same healthy benefits as its high-intensity cousins. Science has shown without a shadow of a doubt that walking regularly raises HDL cholesterol and reduces LDL cholesterol simultaneously. On top of all that, it lowers your risk of obesity, having heart disease, a wider waist circumference, high cholesterol, and high blood pressure, in addition to reducing your chances of suffering from cancer, depression, osteoporosis, type 2 diabetes, and a running list of other major and minor health concerns.

Believe in what's truly possible. Finally, I want you to be reasonable about what you expect from being active on a regular basis. A lot of times, it's not the workout programs that fail us, but our expectations of them. Look, if you're hoping to see instant results from exercise, you're not going to find them. Nearly all the changes I mentioned in this section don't happen overnight, but they do happen.

I'm saying this now because when it comes to most people's goals, weight loss is one of the most popular. Even with everything in balance—your diet and your activities, in particular—your body is only capable of losing an average of one to two pounds a week when you're doing it the healthy way (which is how you'll be doing it following the advice in this book). If you're losing more than that, you're not eating enough, you're overworking yourself, and those extra few pounds you're losing won't be fat but more likely lean muscle tissue (which will cause your metabolism to slow down) and water (from dehydration).

That said, remind yourself that the results you want for yourself are coming—but they decide the pace.

Believe—In Who and What's Around You

When others write your eulogy—what do you want them to say about you?

I know that might sound morbid, but I'm serious. What words would you hope to see? What's the impact you want to make on the world and those around you? Because whether you like it or not, your actions right now will decide how you'll be remembered, no matter what you wish for.

Do you want them to say you just stayed home and did nothing? Do you want to be remembered just for the facts (they were born in this town, worked here, lived there), or do you want to be celebrated for being a good friend?

I've never understood anyone who liked to brag that they were a loner as if that was a good thing. All that ever tells me is that person doesn't fully understand how necessary it is to socialize and communicate on a regular basis, especially with those who support you.

What's my point? If you've been paying more attention to the sections related to your diet, your activities, and yourself—but skimming the sections related to "who and what's around you"— this section is for you. According to research,[17] the relationships you build and nurture play a significant role in your physical and mental health, your health behavior, and even your risk of mortality. That's why I need you to believe in the importance of investing in the relationships in your life, especially if you want to lead a healthier, longer life.

Believe that friends keep your stress in check. Whenever you stress out, your body secretes cortisol—a hormone that raises your blood sugar and blood pressure, so you have energy to either fight or run from whatever's stressing you out. But when you're always in that state, that flow of cortisol stays elevated longer than necessary, putting your health at risk of developing a series of conditions.

The short-term damage is bad enough, ranging from insomnia, headaches, acne and eczema, fatigue, and digestive problems to more serious issues, including chronic pain and high blood pressure, and slowing down your metabolism. Long-term chronic stress can even lead to depression, anxiety, fertility issues, heart disease, weight gain,[18] and gastrointestinal problems, including ulcers and gastroesophageal reflex disease (GERD).

Even though your friends might stress you out sometimes— we're all human, right?—having friends is a powerful tool that keeps your stress levels in check.[19] Part of the reason has to do with feeling more secure, less depressed, and having support during difficult times. But even something as simple as getting a hug from a buddy[20] or laughing with your friends has been shown to release feel-good endorphins (oxytocin, in particular) and significantly lower cortisol and other stress hormones (such as epinephrine) that can negatively impact your health.

Believe that friends make you physically healthier. What exactly is the secret behind why having quality friends improves your physical health and well-being? Is it because they encourage us to stick with healthier habits, as well as point out the bad ones pulling us down we may be trying to ignore? Is it the tagalong factor, knowing we always have an exercise partner or somebody to hit the ball across the court to? It really doesn't matter what the connection is, only that research has proven having friendships pays off.

If you don't think that friends help you stay healthy, research has shown that those with close, meaningful connections experience a lower risk of a variety of different medical issues, including high blood pressure, cardiovascular disease, obesity, and even cancer. There's even evidence that staying social may lower inflammation in your body, which could lead to stroke, arthritis, and heart disease.[21]

Believe that friends make you mentally strong. The benefits of developing and maintaining quality friendships go way beyond preventing depression, anxiety, and other issues that can affect your mental health. Maintaining friendships has been shown to prevent mental decline by improving your memory,[22] boosting brain power,[23] and even helping to ease how you respond to pain.[24]

Having someone's ear to bend—friends who listen to what's on our minds—may also have a lot to do with keeping our cognitive abilities sharp long-term. Research has shown that people who feel supported through active listening (in addition to receiving advice from others and emotional support) are more resilient to cognitive diseases, including Alzheimer's and other forms of dementia.[25]

Believe that friends help you live longer. Because of all the physical and mental benefits that having strong relationships can bring, researchers have shown that having a strong social network lowers your risk of premature death even more than diet and exercise alone. In fact, it's estimated that having healthy social ties may give you a 50 percent chance of living an average of seven and a half years longer, according to a meta-analysis of 148 studies.[26]

Starting the process of staying social earlier than later also makes a major difference on your lifespan. New research has shown that women with stronger social connections in their forties and fifties are more protected against chronic health conditions as they age, including osteoporosis, cancer, heart disease, diabetes, and chronic obstructive pulmonary disease (COPD).[27] Point being, not only do friends make our lives more fun and worth living—they extend our lives so we can have even more fun in the process.

Believe—In Yourself

Back when I was nineteen, for some unknown reason, somehow—my grip changed. You see, when you first take up tennis, you play with what's known as a Continental grip (basically, you hold the racquet like you're using a hammer, with your palm parallel to the strings of the racquet). I use a semi-western grip (if you're right-handed, picture rotating your wrist to the right *before* grabbing that hammer, so your palm is slightly underneath the handle). Most pros tend to use a semi-western grip because, as Goldilocks might say, it's "just right." It's easier to produce top spin, you can hit flat—you can do everything. But for some reason, my grip started slipping even more and rotated into what they call a Western grip (where your palm is completely underneath the handle). You'll see some extreme players use that grip, but very few pros use it because all they can play is loopy top spin—playing fast shots is much harder for them.

I still to this day don't know how it happened, but it definitely isn't the way you want to play tennis and be great on any surface, let me tell you. But I knew that if I had kept the habit, my game would've suffered because I was constantly shanking balls. So, I ended up having to work on changing my grip back midseason—and it was so incredibly painful. It took about two months of just sticking with the process before it was all over with, and there were days when I honestly didn't think I could do it—but I eventually did, and it proved to me that if I set my mind to something, I can accomplish it.

I've had a few injuries where I thought to myself, "Wow, I don't know how I'm going to make it through all this." But every time, by believing in the process and, most importantly, in myself—the expected results came over time. It wasn't quick, and most things worthwhile typically never are, but when you learn to trust the process—when you learn to believe in yourself and understand how your thoughts ultimately decide your actions—that's when you have the best chance of forging long-term habits, learning to stay the course, and achieving success.

Believe by expecting success after failure. One time when I was coming back from an injury, I wasn't quite where I needed to be. It was so hard and frustrating that anytime I would miss a shot, negative thoughts would start to creep in. In those moments, each time I failed, I'd remember all the other times I had failed before that. Suddenly, flashbacks of other times when the ball didn't make it over the net or I had missed a shot would pop up.

But what I was doing in those moments was anticipating a failure **that hadn't even happened yet**.

I'm sure this happens to you just as often as it happens to me, but when you really look at it, all that's really occurring in those moments are thoughts. Thoughts that you actually have control over.

When I first realized this, I decided that instead of anticipating my failures when I would make a mistake, I would anticipate my successes. After any flub or misstep, instead of saying, "I should've made that shot because I made it in practice," I retrained my mind to say, "What if I make the next shot? What if I win the next point?"

On the court, I called it "Reset, Reload, Recharge."

- I **reset** my thoughts right after failure by just letting go of whatever the mistake was (missing the shot, for example).
- I **reload** by reminding myself what it is I want to accomplish (making the shot).
- I **recharge** by starting over, positioning my body, and focusing on the task at hand (preparing myself to make the shot).

It's about allowing yourself to be all that you can be at that very moment—and that starts with your thoughts. And the more you practice this process, the more it becomes second nature. You literally retrain your mind in a way that minimizes stress, anxiety, and disappointment, and instead replaces these with hope, self-assurance, and excitement.

Believe in the power of visualization. If you believe it—you will become it. But if you don't believe in visualization, ask yourself: Of all the pessimistic people you know—how many are living the best life possible in your opinion? I'm willing to bet very few, if any, and that's because visualization also works in reverse.

A pessimist expects bad things to happen, and by spending too much time thinking negative thoughts, a lot of their actions, patterns, and habits become negative as well. Staying pessimistic only reinforces those negative behaviors so they stick and become easier overtime, which then causes the person to become even more pessimistic.

It's a vicious cycle they can't get out of, but it's a cycle that starts in their head because they put that negativity in there. Whatever you reinforce—whatever you feel and think—is what you'll eventually do and become. So, if the goal is to experience more positive actions, patterns, and habits, doesn't it just make sense to make sure that whatever you're thinking and feeling is positive instead of negative?

So, when I say visualize, I'm not expecting you to do anything too extreme. Just closing your eyes and visualizing what you wish to achieve is all it takes. But to get more from it, keep the following tips in mind:

- **Imagine the win from start to finish.** Think about every step and every action you need to make to succeed at whatever it is you want to accomplish, then picture yourself doing each of them without making a single mistake.
- **Don't worry about time.** Just closing your eyes for a minute or two is better than nothing.
- **Anything counts.** I don't just visualize a successful performance on the court but also before a meeting, before exercise, even before sitting down to eat a healthy meal. Feel free to visualize for any situation you want to succeed with.
- **Don't limit yourself.** Don't just visualize once a day. Try it at any point of the day as often as possible.

Believe by remembering what you love now was once something new. Sometimes we may settle for the positive things already in our lives, or worse, let nerves get the better of us and stop believing that we need to try new things. That's why, if you ever get to a point where you feel content with not exploring new options, that you've found your fair share of healthy things and don't need to grow or STRIVE any further, I want you to immediately do this:

Take a few minutes and make a quick list of anything you've ever done and everyone in your life right now whom you appreciate and enjoy. I'm talking about whatever and whoever made or makes you happy over the course of your lifetime.

I'm not expecting you to write down every single moment or person, but put a few things down on paper so you have something in front of you. Because most of the things you wrote down—that short list of experiences, activities, and individuals you can't imagine your life being without right now—were, at one point, never a part of your world at all. Until, of course, you made the choice to let them in.

Having the best life possible means being willing to actively and constantly look for new and different experiences, as well as seek out more positive people—but that only happens if you're willing to put yourself out there as often as possible. For all you know, your favorite fruit, vegetable, meal, exercise, activity, or even friend—things or people that could make your journey toward the best life possible even easier—are still out there. So put yourself out there by remembering that what you adore right now was once unknown too.

CHAPTER 9

INSPIRE

Inspiration can come from anywhere, but the biggest slipup most people make is sitting around waiting for inspiration to come to them instead of actively seeking it out. Worse yet, once someone finds something inspiring, they tend to stick with it well past its expiration date.

Here's something very few people know about me. Every single time I won a major championship, I was inspired by something new. Something completely different from the last time I competed—and that was by design. The reason? Because your mind is way smarter than you give it credit for.

It works like this: No matter how inspired you might be to change your lifestyle for the better, that "muse" can quickly become mundane—a bit *too* familiar—when you least expect it. So, if you don't change it up—and I'm talking about changing your source of inspiration as often as possible—your mind isn't shy about eventually telling you flat out: "I already know about that, so what else do you have to keep me wanting to move forward?"

I've always needed to look for new inspirations to help me reach that next level in every single area of my life. It's the fuel that propels you, opens your eyes to your capabilities, and makes you feel as if there are no limitations to what is possible for yourself. It's the secret sauce missing from every lifestyle program I've ever seen. The one thing that—when you're smart enough to seek out inspiring things continually—makes it so easy to not only stick to your health and wellness goals but changes them from things you *have* to do into things you *want* and *need* to do.

When you're inspired, I mean genuinely inspired, nothing can stop you—because you won't let anything get in the way of your goals. But surprisingly, it doesn't take much. For me, it's sometimes been as simple as finding a particular phrase or motto that drove me at critical moments to find more strength or focus harder. Other times, I found it by listening to others' stories of inspiration or by trying a different way of doing something whenever something felt repetitive and boring. The key is giving your mind and body new cues to be a jumping-off place for inspiration.

Inspire—The Right Way

'll admit, finding inspiration isn't always easy for some. But that's because often we sort of get inside our own heads too much trying to figure out what exactly will inspire us. In this section, I'll give you a variety of different ways you can add inspiration to your daily life. Because inspiration is personal, I'm 100 percent certain you're going to find a few other ways on your own that work best for you. Either way, keep these strategies in mind:

It doesn't have to be uniquely yours. Sometimes we're looking for inspiration to be personalized, like focusing on something your parents might've said to you as a kid, or wearing a certain good-luck charm when you work out for inspiration because it's something special to you. Don't get me wrong. When you can find sources of inspiration that are deeply personal, it can be powerful. But if you spend too much time waiting around to try to find them if they aren't easily seen or present, then you're missing out on fueling yourself.

That said, look, this section is filled with different ways to inspire yourself that aren't yours—they're mine. And that's fine so long as a few of them inspire you. That's all that really matters. So instead of wasting too much energy trying to find the *perfect* thing that inspires you, don't be afraid to ask around to find out what inspires others to see what might stick.

It doesn't have to be monumental. Even the tiniest of things can make a massive impact in your motivation. Something as simple as a word—STRIVE, for example (just saying!)—might be all you need to remember or write down so you can see it to stay inspired all day long. Point being, don't worry about the size of the inspiration and trust your senses instead.

Inspiration always has a shelf life—always. Like I said earlier, what used to move me before a championship was different every year by design. Were there times when I considered sticking with the same inspiration as the season before because it worked well for me? Once or twice, but I understood that if I didn't find something new, then that source of inspiration was always going to be less uplifting and encouraging. So even if something works today, don't be afraid to change it when you feel it's not working to spur you on in the same way it did when you first discovered it.

Inspire—Your Diet

How exactly do you find inspiration to eat healthier? The source can come from so many places, but what inspires you? Only you can answer that—but I can give you some pointers that might work for you.

For me, oftentimes I'll just remind myself that when I'm eating unhealthily, I could be using that same amount of time and energy to eat healthy. That the effort of trying to decide what flavor ice cream I want or which junky food will satisfy me could've been spent looking for or preparing something that's better for me. I remind myself that it's really just a moment when I'm eating these foods—a moment. And when that's over, the effects of what I just had are going to be sticking around a lot longer. The real question becomes, *Will I be happy once those effects finally rear their ugly heads?*

It's a mental game for me, and I spend a lot of time thinking, "Okay, I'm going to eat this right now, but in twenty minutes, am I even going to remember this meal? Is that moment going to last as long as the time I might have to spend in the gym working out to burn off those calories—or the many moments of guilt I might feel afterward?" I'm not saying I can talk myself into making the best choice all the time, but it definitely reminds me that I can say no.

How will you find inspiration to eat healthier? That's for you to decide, but there are a few motivational maneuvers you can try until you find the one that works in the moment.

Inspire by letting the season guide you. With so many fruits and vegetables to choose from, a fun way to inspire your diet is to let the season decide for you. You can put this inspiring trick to good use by asking local farmers or the produce manager in your supermarket what's in season, then picking those foods first during the short window of time they're available over your usual choices.

For example, I love summer fruit and can't wait for peach season because, when it hits, I'll eat as many as I can until it's over. I'll do the same for other types of fresh produce as well. That doesn't mean I'm not eating anything else, but it helps me rotate the fruits and vegetables I'm eating throughout the year without really thinking about it, so I get a more diverse balance of vitamins and minerals.

Inspire by taking a pic of the perfect meal. Instead of posting pictures of your meals to impress others on social media, take one of your breakfast, lunch, and dinner (as well as every snack) before you eat them, then scroll through those pictures at the end of the day. You may like what you see, but if you don't, figure out what's on your plate that you have the biggest problem with, then push yourself to take a better picture next time.

This inspiration is sort of a contest with yourself to try to beat your own score, so to speak. For example, the next time you have breakfast, look back at your last picture and see if you can create (or choose) a breakfast that beats it by being even better for your body. You can step it up a notch and challenge your friends to see who ate the healthiest meal during the day.

Inspire by exploring every version. Even when we eat healthy, we can get stuck in a rut with certain foods. One way I like to inspire myself is to prepare a vegetable in every possible way for one week, so long as it's healthy. For example, if you like broccoli, have it steamed on Monday, roasted on Tuesday, sautéed in olive oil on Wednesday, grilled on Thursday, baked on Friday, raw on Saturday, then pick your favorite way of making it on Sunday.

Why the same vegetable over the same week? Isn't it important to have a mixture of different types of vegetables? It is, and I just want you to try this inspirational trick occasionally to get over the point that each style of cooking brings out a uniquely different flavor from a vegetable. That way, the next time you're bored with eating a particular food a certain way or feel resistant to even trying a food you think you hate, you can use this as inspiration to remind yourself that you have other options in terms of how you prepare it.

Inspire by mastering measurements. Knowledge is power, and often, our intentions of eating better are honorable—it's just that we're not as good at calculating how much we've eaten. The trick is knowing what an average serving size is without calling attention to yourself. I mean, if you're fine with pulling out teaspoons and measuring cups every meal, have at it. But if you want to spare yourself the looks but still have control over what you eat, you just need to know what's what when it comes to certain standard ways to eyeball your food:

- A serving of cheese (one oz.) is the same size as two pairs of dice.
- A serving of chicken, fish, or meat (cooked, three oz.) is the same size as a deck of cards or the palm of your hand (if you're a woman).
- A serving of nuts, chips, or pretzels (one oz.) is about one handful.
- A serving of vegetables or fruit—as well as one cup serving of cooked rice or whole-grain pasta—is around the size of a tennis ball.
- A serving of oils, fats, or butter (one tsp.)—as well as a single serving of salad dressing—is around the size of the tip of your thumb.
- A serving of salad is roughly the size of an open cupped hand.
- A serving of peanut butter (two tbsp.) is the same size of a Ping-Pong ball.

These are just the basics, but if you really want to inspire your diet, figure out how you can gauge other foods that you typically eat (both healthy and unhealthy) by measuring out one serving, then figuring out what it looks like. Could you pour it all into your hand? Is it the size of your finger? Once you have those rough measurements in your head, you'll be inspired to eat the right amount of that food the next time.

Inspire by replacing meals with memories. If you're choosing certain unhealthy foods because they remind you of your childhood or a happier time in your life, then try putting down the food you're about to eat and focusing on that memory instead. In fact, I want you to do the exact opposite and grab something extremely healthy. Then as you eat it, just settle in with that memory.

If you have pictures, letters, mementos, or anything related to that memory, break them out—or reach out to anyone who shared that memory with you. The more often you do this, the more likely you'll be to separate the actual moment that's really making you happy from the meal that's making you unhealthy.

Inspire your aqua habits. Many of the tricks I've already shared (such as infusing your water) can inspire you to drink more. However, there are still a few other tactics you can "set and forget" that can help you effortlessly hit that target number of sixty-four ounces a day without really thinking about it too much.

Put a straw in it. For some weird reason, most people tend to take larger sips and reach for their drink more often when using one.

Be a glass-half-full type of person. Waiting for your glass to be empty before refilling it can sometimes increase your chances of not drinking as often. How? Because some people will look at their half-empty glass and think, "I'm doing a good job!" and then they sort of leave it that way. Instead, as soon as your glass or water bottle hits the halfway point, immediately refill it. Chances are you'll probably drink some of it on the way to the sink or refrigerator. But more importantly, always having a full container makes you more likely to remember to drink.

Have a drink in every room. Well, maybe not every room, but who really stays in one room of their house all day long? Instead, put a glass of water in various parts of your house (the kitchen, your living room, your bedroom, the basement, etc.). As you move from room to room, stop and take a few sips before doing whatever it is you went there to do.

Let the clock time your chugs. Something we all do throughout the day is check the time, so make a deal with yourself to always take a sip every time you do it. If that's not your thing, pick any activity that you know you're guilty of doing at least fifty-plus times a day (checking the weather, looking at your inbox, scrolling through social media, whatever) and then only allow yourself to do it *after* you've taken at least one to three sips of water.

Inspire—Your Activities

You don't have to go far to find inspiration in your activities. Sometimes, it can be as easy as relocating yourself someplace else, reflecting on what you're already great at, or even realizing that others around you are already showing you new roads to travel if you know where to look.

Inspire by changing the scenery. Have you ever driven down the same road repeatedly, so many times that you thought you knew everything there was to see along the way? And then one day, you find yourself in the passenger seat for a change, and even though you're going down the exact same road you've driven hundreds of times—the journey seems a little bit different somehow?

Even when you're not tweaking your workouts or activities to keep your muscles guessing, it's still important to experiment with other ways to make whatever you're doing a little more interesting, inspirational, and fun. So many things are under our control—things that really don't take any extra energy to set in motion—but only if you're aware of what to do and how to take advantage of the simple, little difference makers, such as:

- *The time of day:* If you're typically active in the morning, try the afternoon or evening and vice versa. Just the difference in sunlight, your energy levels, or a different mix of people exercising around you will make the same workout feel different.

- *Move a few feet over:* Some people like to use the same piece of cardio equipment, be in the same row of an exercise class, or stand in a specific place when they're performing certain exercises. Instead, make a point when possible to step away from whatever spot you typically gravitate toward.

- *Test drive someplace else:* Even if you already have a gym membership, try a different place on for size.

- *Switch rooms—or rearrange one:* If you exercise at home, sweat it out somewhere else besides your go-to spot. And if you're stuck in that spot, just turn around 180°. Changing your view by even a few degrees can keep your brain from being bored by feeling *just* a little different.

- *Take it outside:* I do this every chance I get, but not just because it makes me feel good and more energized. Research shows that being around green space (trees and grass) not only reduces stress but lowers your risk of developing many serious health issues, including high blood pressure, type 2 diabetes, and cardiovascular disease.[1]

- *Consider your colors:* When possible, avoid exercising in poorly lit rooms or those painted brown, black, gray, or gold, since dark lighting and some colors can leave you feeling more relaxed.

Instead, choose a well-lit spot or rooms painted with brighter colors—such as yellow, red, orange, or light blue—all of which trigger alertness and can make you feel more energized.

Inspire by being active when it's least convenient. Life doesn't always make it easy to exercise on a regular basis, does it? Even when we tell ourselves we're going to exercise or be active, let's say, three or four times a week for at least thirty minutes, that's when life doesn't really care what we told ourselves and makes it difficult to stick to our promises.

But what often decides whether a person stays healthy for life is whether they can roll with the punches. Whether or not, when things get crazy busy and it's not as easy to exercise, they figure out a way to move things around and make time to be active, no matter what.

At certain points over the decades I've practiced, life stepped in and tested my commitment to the sport or myself. In fact, life probably gets in the way more than it doesn't. The only difference is that during those moments when the last thing I wanted to do was train or exercise, I did it anyway because I knew that progress takes persistence. I had to find inspiration on days that were determined to work against the plans I might've had for myself in those moments.

Now it's your turn. Can you find that inspiration when life makes things inconvenient? Try planning one of your workouts during the worst part of your week. Seriously, look ahead, see which day is your absolute worst, then pencil that workout somewhere between it all.

I'm not going to sweet-talk this. Will it be fun that day? Probably not. Are you going to want to pull your hair out trying to juggle everything? No doubt. But at the end of the day, you'll have proved to yourself that when you *want* to, nothing can "stop" you from finding the time to be active. That way, the next time life doesn't make it easy—you'll find the inspiration to pull off what you used to say was impossible.

Inspire by adding to your strengths. What would you say is an exercise or activity that you're pretty good at? Don't worry, you don't have to be a master at it because this isn't about comparing your skills against anyone. Instead, I just want you to think about something that you're not half bad at.

Look, it doesn't matter whether you consider yourself uncoordinated or out of shape (for now) or if you're a complete novice when it comes to working out or being active. Even the most "exercise awkward" person has at least one thing they've tried to do— one activity, one exercise, one stretch, one yoga pose, whatever it is—that they realized they could do. It will be something that someone else might struggle with—but not them.

So what is it for you? And if you don't know, ask others where they believe your strengths lie. Just know that all you need is *one* example of being good at something, because the fact that you already have at least one is proof of what you can do—and that you're capable of adding one more.

That's why from there, your goal will be to add *one* more to that list of strengths—whether that's trying to be good at one more activity, one more exercise, one more stretch, one more yoga pose. That new strength can come from any direction, and it doesn't matter how long it takes, so long as you're moving in the direction—and putting in the necessary effort—to improve that number by one.

Inspire by being a silent observer. You may never know where the next big thing to inspire you when it comes to exercise or being active will come from, or when it will even happen—but that doesn't mean you can't change the odds to be in your favor by seeking it out yourself.

Athletes do this all the time by watching the games, matches, and competitions of other athletes to look for pointers on form and execution. Looking for the little details of what someone else might be doing to perform at their best. I do it all the time, replaying not just matches of my own to see how my opponent was able to get the jump on me at certain moments, but other players' matches as well. Any smart athlete will admit that they don't keep blinders on or ignore what everybody else is doing—they keep their eyes wide open to what might be helpful to them down the road.

Just because you're not a competitive athlete doesn't mean you can't do the same thing. On days when you're giving your body a rest from activity or exercise (since I wouldn't want you to be distracted from your own workout on days that you're active), try going to the gym anyway and just find a spot to watch from for a while.

- You could focus on a specific station to see how people may use it differently.
- You could focus on a specific person who seems to reflect your own goals, and just observe their entire program (their tempo, the exercises they choose, how many reps and sets they do, their form, etc.).
- You could focus on the free-weight area to see who might be doing some interesting exercise that you've never seen before.

Most of the time, you might be observing someone who knows less than you, but other times, it may be someone who knows more. In that case, don't be afraid to walk up and ask them (after they've finished their workout and only if appropriate) why they chose to do whatever it was that intrigued you. Who knows? You may discover a better or new way to do what you've been doing to get in shape—or something you never thought of trying until that very day.

Inspire—Who and What's Around You

What's the expression—a rising tide lifts all boats? Being a positive force around others by encouraging them and staying optimistic—inspiring them to pursue their goals and reminding them that they can do it—not only improves their lives but generally makes those around you do the same for you.

In certain sections of the book (such as the "Appreciate," "Enrich," and "Soothe" chapters), I showed you a few different ways you can support others, but inspiration can take many forms, some of them not as direct as others. Meaning sometimes you can inspire those around you without ever speaking to them—or even knowing them—just by acting a particular way or being a certain type of person.

Think about it: Of the people who have inspired you, how many know the effect they had on you? Earlier in the book, I asked you to **appreciate those who got you here** because there's always at least one person responsible for your life running down the right track, all because of something they said or did that inspired you, even if they have no idea they had that effect on you.

Well, now it's your turn to potentially be that person for someone else. Some of the suggestions I'm proposing are a little more direct but others are just about attitude. Because when you're positive, you never know who you're going to inspire. But when you're negative, you may never realize how many enemies you're making or people you're turning away. The impact you make on the world matters because we all make one—but what we give, we also get back.

Inspire by being up—even when you're down. When we're miserable and going through a tough week, don't have enough free time, or might not be feeling our best, it can be so hard to be upbeat. But it's so important to stay positive even when you're not in that headspace because those moments don't last forever. When they pass, they're gone and we sort of forget about them, right? But what's not forgotten is how you might've negatively impacted others by letting yourself linger in all that negativity.

Another reason to stay cheerful and not let being miserable ruin the moment is how it can help you persevere the next time. How we act and behave in those moments oftentimes decides how we'll act and behave the next time we're upset. Think of it like "muscle memory." The more you train yourself to stay positive when things turn negative, the easier it becomes to automatically look at every bad time that comes your way with a positive attitude.

If you're having one of those rough moments in your life right now, remind yourself that you've moved on from moments even rougher than this and overcame them. Think about the last time you were worried about something that's no longer a concern. Focus on the fact that a month from now, you're probably not even going to remember this moment, so stay positive as you go through it, not just because you'll inspire others but because it will help you push through that moment much faster. Allow yourself to remember that moments are nothing more than moments, and sure, sometimes you can't change your circumstance, but you can change your attitude—and oftentimes, your attitude can change your circumstance.

Inspire by rewarding someone else for your successes. In the "Enrich" chapter of this book, I suggested ways to reward yourself for a job well done, whether by sticking to your diet, exercising a certain number of days a week, or continuing whatever healthy strategy you stuck with. But what would happen if instead of doing something for yourself, you flipped the script and gave that reward to someone you cared about instead? I'm talking about making a promise to somebody that they will get some sort of reward—*if* you stay on a healthy path for a certain amount of time.

What I love about this way to inspire is that it works on so many levels:

- It makes you accountable to somebody, so that even if you *might've* considered skipping a day of exercise or eating something unhealthy, it's really hard to blow off what you've set out to do when you know that friend's going to ask about it later.
- That same person becomes your personal cheerleader of sorts, rallying behind you to complete whatever healthy habit you promised you would stick with.
- Finally, watching you stay true to your health goals might get them to ask questions about what you're doing or could inspire them to try to do whatever it is you're doing as well.

Inspire by being the dependable one. No one wants to be known as the person who can't be counted on. Sure, most of us probably consider ourselves reliable and always there when needed. But when was the last time you broke a promise to meet up with somebody or help them out? When was the last time someone asked for help and you said, "You know, that sounds great—but let me get back to you on that."

So how does being the dependable one inspire others around you? Easy, because whenever you show someone you're dependable and keep your promises to them, you're building trust with that person. And that goes a long way toward not only strengthening the relationship you have but motivating them to do the same for you down the road.

But that sense of commitment also extends to others who witness your behavior, and even to people you've never met. When you're reliable on a regular basis, you're literally building a reputation for yourself as someone who's honorable—and unfortunately, there aren't many like that in the world. You're setting an example of what's easily possible by just being trustworthy. An example that might not inspire everyone to follow suit, but even if just one person is motivated by your principles, well then—you've just made the world a little better without doing anything but being a reliable friend.

Inspire—Yourself

My sister and I like to joke with each other whenever we see an opportunity we both may want to try but don't want to step on each other's toes. It could be something as simple as seeing the same pair of shoes. If one of us didn't want them, the other will say out of respect, "Do you mind if *I* move on it?"

When it comes to design, I'm always looking for that next new thing, person, thought, or saying that's going to motivate me in one direction or the other. I'm always putting myself in situations that inspire me, and I actually get very upset when I see interior design that's not inspiring—it's weird but true.

It starts with my mindset. I like being pushed, and the best way to be pushed is by people who are being great around you. Those are the ultimate role models of what to do, how to do it, and why to do it. So when I'm not around others like that, I get upset because I know that when those types of people are present, it also makes me better. If I have an idea, I want to see an even better idea because it means that I can do that too.

The world is moving so fast these days that it's not always easy to find inspiration, but it's out there, sometimes right in front of you just waiting for you to see it. That's why when you do get inspired, it's important to "move on it."

I could give you a list of things to do that might inspire you, but what inspires me may not work for you. I could encourage you to travel more, read more, hit a bunch of museums and other culture-packed places, even tell you to just go outside and stare at nature for a while. But when that's not always an option, you can just as well inspire yourself in other ways that don't require a passport or even having to leave your home. No matter where you find inspiration, the only thing that matters is that you move on it—whatever that "it" is for you.

Inspire by removing what no longer moves you. I need to feed my creativity, which is why I'm constantly pinning things up, creating mood boards, watching runway shows, and going to places where I see inspirational objects or things that make me want to be as artistic and expressive. When I do that, thoughts come into my head much easier, and I have a better flow when it comes to design. But when I don't get that opportunity, I get upset. That's why I pay close attention to the things that keep me motivated and creative.

Somewhere close by, there's a piece of inspiration around you that's way past its expiration date. Maybe it's that college diploma on your wall or some trophy you always forget about until you have to dust it. Something that, at one time, may have held meaning and inspired you, but today, just doesn't have that same power over your spirit like it once did. So, ask yourself: Why is it still there? Instead of just taking it down, actively find something new to replace it that truly inspires you.

Inspire by finding a new mantra often. Words can be so inspirational, and maybe there's a phrase you've heard in the past that made such an impact on you that you remind yourself of it often. One that you repeat whenever you're down or doubtful to help you get back up and try again. Or one that you say every morning to start the day in the right mindset, or every night to slow your world down and relax.

I'm guilty of finding certain quotes, mantras, and phrases that helped guide and motivate me through different seasons throughout my career and different moments throughout my life. But I've never stuck with the same one for the entire journey because, as we change and grow, so should the words that once moved you.

I want you to find that phrase for yourself. It doesn't have to be poetic or perfect in any way. You could literally pick a word that you wish you could be right now—happy, energetic, healthier, etc.—run that word through a thesaurus to find other words that match it, then just put the words "I will be," "I am," or "I deserve to be" in front of it. For example:

- I will be *carefree*.
- I am *dynamic*.
- I deserve to be *strong*.

Whether you make your own mantra or find one elsewhere that fits you, say it aloud as often as possible, especially in moments when you need to hear it most, but just recognize that it fits you for the moment. Before that phrase no longer has power over you—before those words coming out of your mouth are just words—find another mantra that drives you even further.

Inspire by wearing what works for you. I like to wear clothes that I know make me feel great about myself, because if you don't feel that way as often as possible—in every possible situation—then you need to do something about it. Even with matches, if I didn't like an outfit or didn't feel my best in it, I would change it—during the match!

I remember when I first started to go to development meetings for my design business. I would go all out and put on a suit because that's what you do to look serious, right? But I never felt confident or creative until I finally realized: "This isn't me—so why am I wearing this?" After that, I started showing up looking like myself—and I was not only free but finally felt confident and creative again.

Look, I get it. I understand the importance of making a good impression. But if you're wearing something that's uncomfortable, you're going to be too busy focusing on all that unpleasantness instead of the task at hand. Instead, finding something that makes you feel good, makes you feel powerful, makes you feel like *you* brings more strength and self-assurance to any situation, no matter what you need to tackle.

Now, everybody's got their own style, so I can't tell you what to wear that will inspire you or what your power colors might be. But if losing weight and getting fitter are part of your agenda, then at least wear clothes that allow you to move freely. Getting the most out of exercise means being able to go through the greatest range of motion with your muscles. If you can't bend, stretch, or reach in any garment just as easily as if you weren't wearing that piece of clothing, find something that offers you a little more flexibility.

Inspire by remembering what really matters. Let's be honest: often what pushes us to get in shape is a moment. Maybe it's to look better for an event, a beach vacation, or any moment where we want to impress others. Or maybe it's making healthier choices because of numbers we didn't like seeing after having a moment with your doctor. But living a healthier lifestyle shouldn't be a moment attached to making certain people jealous or getting others off your back.

Ultimately, I want you STRIVING toward improving your health and wellness not just because you deserve it but because of what *really* comes with that kind of life that you may not even be considering. Instead of attaching a date or number to the healthy actions you're taking, I want you to think about how your life will be better all around—and that whatever health-based successes come from that (losing weight or lowering your cholesterol, for example) are just cherries on a much bigger sundae. From this point forward:

- Don't look at every pound you lose as a means to fitting into some silly dress or pair of pants. Instead, remember every pound lost is an opportunity to do and try more things with your body.
- Don't just look at the numbers that are improving—your blood pressure, blood sugar, cholesterol—as indicators that you're healthier. Instead, remind yourself that keeping those numbers under control not only means living a longer, healthier life but being able to make the most of every single day.
- Forget about the aesthetics and recognize that the fitter you become, the more doors in life open to you by allowing you to experience more things, visit more places, spend more quality time doing the things you love to do—or haven't even yet gotten the chance to do, but soon will—with the people you love.

CHAPTER 10

STRIVE

For as long as I can remember, I have always worked toward a goal—and my spirit and purpose has never changed. Because I feel that no matter where you are in life or how far you've come—it's never the end. There's always more room to grow.

Many people go through life feeling unimportant, incapable, and irrelevant, as if the world doesn't want what they have to offer or say—but that's only because they fail to try. We always have to strive to stay relevant. When you feel irrelevant, I think that is a choice *you* make for yourself, whether consciously or unconsciously—but it is a choice nonetheless. To stay relevant, you continuously need to strive toward something or else you'll never know what you are truly capable of.

In the middle of my tennis career, I did something that surprised (and I guess even scared) a few people around me. I decided to hit the books and finish my degrees in both fashion design and business administration. Most thought I was crazy to do it, and I was repeatedly asked: "Wouldn't it be better to wait until after you stop playing tennis professionally? Isn't it risky to pursue two passions at the same time?"

But I knew back then—as I still do now—that when you're continually learning, you're always growing. And that growth doesn't have to get in the way of other goals you may have for yourself. Instead, it can branch out and boost your other goals. And when you do it right, it can fortify every single part of you and what you do, no matter how many different directions you want to explore.

It's understanding that what we put into our life always helps us get more out of it. Regularly being exposed to something new every chance I get has not only made my life a more fulfilling, healthier, and happier one but, surprisingly, it's made it even easier to concentrate on health and wellness. You would think that adding new things could be distracting, but I firmly believe that when you purposely and consistently add new skills, experiences, and knowledge into your life, it enriches everything else you're presently focused on.

Are your goals different from mine? Sure, they are, but then again, they should be. Because I'm not talking about needing to strive toward being the absolute best in something. In fact, I have a saying, which is *Better—not best—because "best" is just a moment.* I'm talking about going after whatever might bring you joy and make you a happier person tomorrow. I'm talking about waking up every morning excited and energized because you know there's something out there waiting for you—and no one is going to stop you from realizing it.

The reason I insist you always be in a "state of striving" is also because many experts agree that when you're focused on a future goal, it creates purpose. It gives your life meaning and leaves you feeling more fulfilled, experiencing less regret and stress, and ultimately makes you happier.

STRIVE—The Right Way

In this section, I'm going to show you a variety of ways you could rethink what's possible for yourself to open new doors to healthier opportunities and experiences. But to do it right, these tactics should be top of mind:

Never doubt how much you can tackle. Some of the challenges in this section might seem impossible, but I want you to give yourself a little credit. Just the fact that you're here means you're ready for a change in your life. How big of a change and how many changes, well—that's for you to decide. You really must think about how much you can bite off, and I want to encourage you to take a big bite!

Just because STRIVE is a program that lets you do as little or as much as you like, I don't want to encourage you to think, "Hmmm . . . how little can I do to pull this thing off?" Instead, I want you to ask yourself, "How much can I do—and still do well?" And even then, I want you to ask yourself, "Hmm . . . can I go past that a little bit?"

But don't take on more than you can handle. We all know our breaking point, right? And if you don't know yours, it really doesn't take much to figure it out. If at any point as you STRIVE, you feel overwhelmed, anxious, and stressed—then you're standing right in front of it.

There are so many things I want to try, but I've had to recognize that I can't do them all at once. It's entirely fine to have a lot of goals for yourself, but you can't be a jack-of-all-trades. We only have so much capacity to stay on top of what we want to take on, which is why I've always believed in having between three to five goals at most at one time (or for a period of time). It's a standard that successful companies apply to their business and culture, and it's a model that works equally well when integrated into daily life.

That said, the beauty of STRIVE is that you never really have to get to that place. As you'll see in Chapter 11, how much effort you put into the program is up to you. If it ever feels like following these eight actions is way too much, then you're probably pushing yourself harder than you're ready for at the moment. And that's okay, because you'll get there. But until you do, just dial it back a little bit.

Sit back—and enjoy the struggle. When was the last time you heard anybody take pride in—or heard yourself take pride in, for that matter—accomplishing something easy or insignificant? When did you last brag about a task that didn't take up much time or effort? I'm willing to bet you haven't—because nobody ever talks about or remembers the easy wins. No, we remember the big victories—the ones we fought hard for.

I don't know how you're going to STRIVE or what portions of this section you're going to use in your life, but I do know that some will be harder than others—and they will test you. In those moments when you think you've bitten off more than you can chew, step back from it all and recognize that whatever you chose to try might be difficult, but ask yourself if it's doable. Because if it is, then it's worth sticking with it. It may feel like a struggle now, but you must learn to love the battle. Because that battle will lead to more benefits down the line—and give you a greater sense of pride once you win.

STRIVE—With Your Diet

Sometimes, you just need a challenge to give your nutrition a little jumpstart. Nothing so extreme that you can't stick to it, but nothing so easy that it's not even worth the effort.

I'm not talking about attempting some fad diet, because in my world, diet is a four-letter word I never say or do. No, I'm talking about striving toward a nutritional goal that, if pulled off, even if it's just for a short period of time, will not only make you feel a difference but also prove to yourself what you're able to accomplish.

I'll give you an example: Back in 2022, I wanted to get ready for the Oscars because we had been nominated for the movie about my dad (*King Richard*). So I thought, "Okay, what else could I try besides what I already do?" At the time, I was already eating pretty healthy, but after honestly observing my habits, I knew I could stand to cut out some of my snacking. I'm only human, and snacking was still one of my weaknesses, so I decided to challenge myself by staying completely away from snacks throughout the month of January.

Oh, I got teased by my friends and family who used to say in this singsongy way that I was going through my "snack free . . . Janu—erreee!" but I didn't let that stop me. And in the beginning, being honest, it was sooooo hard—especially at night. That's when I would have more free time and always found myself looking in the pantry for snacks. I could have snacks, but they had to be fruits or nuts, and even with that, I only allowed myself a finite amount to eat. But then once January passed, something interesting happened—I had broken myself from snacks altogether!

The thing is, I hadn't even thought about it. It wasn't until the middle of February that I suddenly realized I didn't obsess about snacks anymore. I mean, all my life I had been a snacker. But somehow, I had turned a fun challenge into an unconscious habit—something I wasn't planning on or ever in my life expected to happen.

That's what I want for you. I want you to strive toward something nutritionally, just to see what happens. It doesn't have to be something tricky, difficult, or incredibly game-changing to count. It just has to be something that motivates you. A task with just enough challenge to it that it might seem a little bit impossible to pull off—until you prove it's possible. Because you'll never be quite sure what you're capable of—until you actually try.

Some of these suggested challenges can be tried on for size just for the day, while others might be something you want to STRIVE with continuously for a week, a few weeks, maybe even a month (or just to see how long you can stay committed to it), especially if you really want to see and feel their positive effects long term.

STRIVE to eat a healthy food you've never tried before. I mean, do your research first to make sure you're not being misled about the food being healthy for you. But once you know it is, buy it and try it. If you don't like it, I'm not expecting you to eat the whole thing. But if you do like it, then you've just added another healthy option you can turn to for the rest of your life. How cool is that?

Honestly, what I really love about this STRIVE is that you could do this every day of your life and never run out of options, which proves a point. If you've ever complained that one reason you're not as healthy as you could be is because you really don't like that many good-for-you foods, this challenge will prove that you just haven't explored everything that's out there waiting for you.

STRIVE to pull off as many RDAs as possible. Throughout this book, I mentioned a few recommended daily allowances (RDAs) and daily values of certain nutrients, but that's the thing. We all know some of them because they're thrown at us all the time—the suggested amounts of what to eat (or limits) each day—but when was the last time you *actually* did it? I mean made the effort to focus solely on that number all day, no matter what? Right—me neither.

Truth be told, you don't have to shoot for a specific RDA or Daily Value as much as whatever is usually the standard recommended amount nutritionists vouch for, such as:

- Eating fourteen grams of dietary fiber per one thousand calories. This means roughly twenty-five grams (for women) or thirty-eight grams (for men).

- Limiting your sugar intake to no more than six teaspoons for women (twenty-five grams) or nine teaspoons for men (thirty-six grams) per day.
- Drinking at least sixty-four ounces of water a day.
- Limiting your sodium intake to less than twenty-three hundred milligrams a day.
- Limiting your saturated fat intake to twenty grams a day.

Seriously, there's a recommended amount (or limit) for pretty much every vitamin, mineral, or other important nutrient once you go down this rabbit hole, which is why I won't list them all here. But the ones above are some of the big ones that, when paid attention to, can really pay off some serious dividends health-wise. Try testing yourself with just one to see how long you can do it, or see how many you could pull off in one day. No matter how you play this one, your body always wins.

STRIVE to forsake fried foods for at least a week. I know it's all delicious, but it's also high in saturated fat, clogs your arteries, and raises your risk of hypertension[1] and heart failure, type 2 diabetes,[2] cancer, and even Alzheimer's. Because most people don't eat fried foods every day (and if you do, you really need to do this), try striving away from them for a minimum of seven days to make an impact.

STRIVE to be a serious journalist. Even though I've asked you to write down things you've observed about your diet, I'm talking about taking it to the next level. What that means is literally tracking every morsel and every drop you eat or drink for the day in every possible way, which can sometimes help you understand your eating habits and food choices a lot better.

If you're up for it, here are just a few observations you could jot down (although how detailed you want to get is entirely up to you):

- Where you ate—and the time of day.
- How hungry you were (before and after) on a scale of 1 to 10.
- What your energy was (before and after) on a scale of 1 to 10.
- What your mood was (before and after).
- The exact amount or number of calories, protein, fat, and carbohydrates in each meal/snack.

STRIVE to find the healthiest thing on the menu. I love going out to eat, who doesn't? But instead of scrolling down the menu thinking with your stomach, strive to find the absolute best thing to eat for your health—and then order it over anything else.

I love this challenge for several reasons: One, it boosts your awareness about what you *could* be eating instead of always ordering your indulgences. Two, it might make you aware that certain places may not have your best interests at heart, especially if you struggle to find anything healthy. Finally, you could realize it was never about the food that made it your favorite place to go and that it was more about the people or the atmosphere.

Want to take it to another level? Go to whatever drawer you've thrown all your takeout menus (I know you have one) and take a few minutes figuring out what the top three healthiest choices are. That way, the next time you find yourself having to order out, you'll be more likely to buy something that's good for you instead of just listening to what your growling stomach may be craving.

STRIVE for four—or fewer—ingredients. This one takes some planning, and it definitely requires a little reading on your part, but I want you to try to avoid eating and drinking anything with more than four ingredients.

This STRIVE is like the suggestion I offered in the "Enrich—Your Diet" section (where I asked you to choose foods with fewer ingredients), but takes it a step further because, when you limit yourself to foods that have four or fewer ingredients, it starts to really pare down your options.

With this one, STRIVE with four to start (trust me, that alone will be challenging), and then if that becomes easy, taper it down to three, then two, then eventually one. At that point, you're literally eating nothing but foods in their original state because you'll have no choice.

The great news is that even though I don't know what foods you're going to choose. Whatever you grab is more than likely going to be much healthier than anything you might've otherwise eaten that day. Whatever you eat or drink, you'll be getting it in a much purer form than it's typically presented, which means it's more likely to be richer in nutrients and free of any manmade ingredients.

STRIVE for an all-water day. It's almost a little too easy to "drink" your calories during the day instead of getting them through your food. And if you're not careful, all those glasses start to add up. But that's the big thing most people focus on—the extra calories. What I think is even worse is how you may be depriving your body of nutrients (beyond H_2O of course).

Most of the beverages we turn to—juice, coffee, soda, energy drinks—are typically lacking in fiber, protein, and healthy fats unless you're making a protein drink, vegetable smoothie, or some type of nutrient-rich drink. That's why I love the challenge of an occasional all-water day.

For one, if you're typically drinking a certain number of calories each day, wouldn't you rather spend those calories on something to eat instead? Two, because most drinks tend to be sweetened in some way, you'll also most likely be taking in less sugar as well. Finally, and this is for those calorie counters out there, your body burns more calories breaking down the food you eat compared to what you drink. Eating more of your daily calories instead of drinking them keeps your metabolism revving a little higher as a side benefit, which your waistline will appreciate.

STRIVE to eat a rainbow. Sometimes I like to make things fun in a crazy way, where I might strive to eat something green at every meal for a week. Sort of like a "green challenge," where it could be a green apple, a pepper, kale, whatever—it just can't be the same green fruit or vegetable twice in one day.

Other times, I might strive to eat a different color every day of the week (by having a red day, then a blue day, then an orange day after that, etc.). Or if I feel up to it, I might try to have all the colors in every meal and snack throughout the day.

Why would I ask you to put yourself through that? Because every fruit and vegetable has its own unique and diverse balance of phytochemicals and phytonutrients inside it. By eating every possible color (or at least targeting the following five color groups), you'll end up absorbing a wider range of flavonoids, carotenoids, anthocyanins, betalains, and other body-beneficial compounds. Here are the five color groups to strive for:

- **Purple/blue:** black raspberries, turnips, eggplant, purple asparagus, purple cabbage, purple carrots, purple kale, endives, Concord grapes, blackberries, blueberries, purple peppers, black olives, elderberries, plums, figs.
- **Green:** spinach, sprouts, kale, broccoli, broccoli rabe, Swiss chard, artichokes, bok choy, kiwis, limes, green peas, avocados, green apples, green grapes, honeydew melon, asparagus, mustard greens, zucchini, turnip greens, arugula, snow peas.
- **Red:** red cabbage, cherries, blood oranges, red bell pepper, red pears, red apples, strawberries, watermelon, red onions, radishes, red potatoes, cranberries, tomatoes, red lettuce, beets, rhubarb.
- **Yellow/orange:** apricots, carrots, cantaloupe, oranges, mangoes, butternut squash, yellow and orange peppers, lemons, sweet

potatoes, pumpkin, pineapples, tangerines, nectarines, papayas, peaches, rutabaga, yellow summer squash, yellow tomatoes.
- **White/light green:** parsnips, cauliflower, bananas, white nectarines, white peaches, ginger, garlic, onions, shallots, mushrooms, napa cabbage, kohlrabi, leeks, and squash.

STRIVE to go as sugar-free as possible. It's not just about the excess pounds eating too much sugar puts on that can lead to diabetes, cancer, high blood pressure, and osteoarthritis, among other issues. It's not even about how it raises your risk of heart disease and kidney stones, causes inflammation, and even messes with your cholesterol by raising your LDL (the bad stuff) and lowering your HDL (the good stuff). No, going sugar-free is about gaining back control of your body.

Just like snacks, I've had the same love-hate experience with sugar. I would spend long periods of time not eating it. I remember once after playing a team competition for the USA, they had candy afterward. I thought, "We won! I'll splurge!" Then immediately after, it felt like I had a hangover. My hands swelled, I felt completely exhausted—it was so intense. But it was a reminder of the power sugar had over me—and that I get to decide if it stays in control.

To do it right, when I say sugar-free, I'm referring to shying away from added sugars. (You'll see what percentage of added sugar is in the food you're eating right on the nutritional label.) Naturally occurring sugars (which are the type you'll find in fruits, vegetables, whole grains, and most dairy products) are okay because at least those foods offer more nutrients and/or fiber and don't raise your blood sugar levels quite as high.

Another reason I love this strive so much is that it really opens your eyes to where sugar hides. Trust me, you may find it virtually impossible to pull this off depending on which foods you regularly eat. And that's just it. It forces you to not only steer clear of what's harmful to your body, but it challenges you to satisfy that sweet tooth in a way that doesn't involve sugar, opening your world to things you otherwise may not have tried before.

STRIVE—In Your Activities

Growing up, my dad always stressed trying something new every chance we got. It wasn't all about tennis. He celebrated and encouraged us to explore other options beyond the game, and I can't stress enough how that was such a great and positive mentality to be raised with.

When I say "activities" for this one, I mean *anything* goes. I'm not just talking about what you do in your leisure time but also possibilities at work or with your side hustle, or ways to further your education. It could be any area of your life where you could be trying something new (or it could even be something you already do but with a fresher perspective).

It doesn't matter what you love to do right now, or what you happen to be great at. It's still important to seek out different activities and new ways of building upon whatever you're currently doing as you become healthier and fitter.

Because when you do, it reminds you and those around you how you're far from a one-trick pony. That you're much more than any one-dimensional persona others may think of you. That you're physically able to bring that same fighting spirit you show in whatever it is others know you for—into anything and everything you decide to set your mind to.

STRIVE by shooting for the impossible. Write down a few activities you've never done before, not because there was no time to do them but simply because you never had much interest in them or just never thought you could pull them off. Activities that never in your wildest dreams could you imagine ever finding their way on your to-do list.

They don't have to be extreme. Maybe it's finally signing up for tennis or dance lessons, trying CrossFit, learning how to mountain bike, or running a 5K or half-marathon. Whatever you write down honestly doesn't even have to be anything you've always wanted to try—it could be just something you're intrigued by. But once you have that short list of activities—this list of things you thought were impossible—pick one and make it possible.

But here's the thing—I don't care how well you do. It's not about crushing whatever you put on that list. It doesn't matter if you're the worst student in the class or you come in last place. The fact that you tried something you wrote down as impossible for *you* to do automatically makes you a winner. And who knows? You may find out you're a natural at something you never expected to be.

STRIVE by evolving your cardio. So, you found a cardiovascular activity that you absolutely love to do? One that, no matter what, you can see yourself doing for the rest of your life, or at least for as long as your body will let you? I know that feeling, and I'm thrilled for you, but here's a question for you: Is it possible to somehow build upon that activity? In other words, what's another possible version of what you enjoy that could make it more of a challenge?

For example, if you love to run, consider trying sprints for a day or running on the beach. Are you a walker? Then maybe take things off-road and turn that walk into a hike. Are you a mountain biker? Then switch to road riding, and if you're already cycling on roads, head to the trails instead. The point is, look for a way to take what you love to do in a slightly different direction to make it more challenging for your body—and more interesting for your mind.

STRIVE by trying every evolution of an exercise. For the most part, when it comes to building lean muscle through resistance training, you can easily get the job done using nothing more than dumbbells and your own body weight—but that doesn't mean you should ever stop there. As you become fitter and more familiar with a certain exercise or move, that's when it's time to explore other ways you can do the same exact exercise but using a different form of resistance, a different grip, even just a different angle to position your body.

For example, remember the dumbbell row exercise I suggested in the "Balance" chapter? There's nothing stopping you from using a kettlebell instead—or a sandbag, resistance bands, or a barbell using two hands. Or the push-up I mentioned? You could easily make it more challenging by putting your feet up on a box instead of keeping them on the floor or by spacing your hands wider than shoulder width apart. Or if you want to go really extreme, you could wear a weighted vest or have someone put a light sandbag over your shoulders.

The point is this: Pretty much every exercise that you're using to build lean muscle has a variety of different versions of itself out there waiting for you to try. So long as you're healthy enough to do them, challenge yourself to find as many different permutations as possible of that exercise that exist—and then try them all.

STRIVE by doing something perfectly. It doesn't matter what you like to do to break a sweat; every activity and exercise has ground rules, right? Somewhere down the line, you learned how to do them step-by-step. Everything from where your feet should be placed, how your arms should be bent, how far to bring the weight down, how to breathe, where your eyes should look as you go—I'm talking about all those things that collectively put it all together.

Most of the time, we learn how to do something to the best of our ability, and then we just do it that way from that point forward. Maybe we pay attention to a few of the details, but chances are that's as far as we take it. But instead of settling, I dare you to try pulling off something perfectly, as if three people were watching with score cards and your only goal is to pull off perfect ten out of tens. Record yourself doing the exercise or activity from as many angles as possible, then give yourself a grade afterward on how perfect your form was. For example:

- If it's an exercise, were your hands and feet in the right spots? How was your posture? Did you go too fast or too slow? Did you always control the weight? Did you bend your arms or legs at the exact angle necessary?
- If it's a specific movement within an activity—like hitting the perfect shot, performing a certain dance movement, running the perfect gait, achieving perfect form when walking—the same rules apply.

What I love about this STRIVE is how it puts you in the zone. Most people assume they're mastering a certain exercise or movement because they've been doing it for a long time. They see results from it, and/or they've never injured themselves doing it. But when you force yourself to literally focus on every single aspect of what you're doing all at once, you'll be surprised how you'll find a slight flaw or two. Tiny flaws that, once fixed, might make the move more comfortable, make it easier to do, or let you achieve more results.

STRIVE—With Who and What's Around You

Even after you've forged your own tight-knit circle of friends, that doesn't mean you shouldn't challenge yourself to work on what you have. How can you do that? By considering things that may push you a little out of your personal comfort zone. When we're honest with others, when we trust them enough to guide us to become better people, when we put a little more of ourselves out there than we typically do, it takes effort, and it can be nerve-racking at times—but it can also be so worth it.

You don't have to go all out to start. Just trying one of these few suggestions could bring a little closure to your life—or bring you closer to someone you care about.

STRIVE to own what you deny. Often, we can't see aspects of who we are because we don't allow ourselves to. So, if you think you're up for it, I want you to ask those closest to you if there's something about yourself that you're not acknowledging. However, it must be something that you could technically work on and improve about yourself. (It can't be anything you have zero control over because that wouldn't be fair.)

Not sure where to start? Or nervous about which direction friends and family might take this open invitation? You can always begin by identifying any area of your life you think could benefit from a little honesty—your personal habits, your relationships, your work ethic, your attitude, etc.—then ask those you trust if there's something you might not be acknowledging in that area that could use a little improvement. To test the waters, make sure they keep it specific to that portion of your life and only offer *one* suggestion so you don't become overwhelmed.

I didn't say it would be easy. This STRIVE is definitely a hard one, so if you would rather dip your toe into the water to start, try asking those same people to define you in a few adjectives—the more examples the better, and no words are off limits. Don't just ask one person but find at least three people who know you best.

Once you have their answers, don't put them on the spot by asking why they chose those words. Instead, take their answers and spend some time alone reflecting on them. After all, this is how other people see you in a nutshell. These are the characteristics that you convey not just to friends but most likely to most people you're around, whether you like it or not.

After you spent some time reflecting, go back to your friends, thank them for caring enough about you to be honest, let them know you're eager to work on any characteristics you weren't necessarily thrilled with, then ask them for suggestions on how to do that. Listen, you may not be ready for what they have to say, but if it's coming from several directions—from people you know genuinely care about you—then remind yourself that whatever they say is coming from a place of love, and something that you need to hear to move forward.

STRIVE to find someone to forgive. None of us are perfect (present company included), and we all make mistakes. Not only that but we all know somebody, at least one person, who probably dropped right off our friend list for screwing up. Can you think about who that person might be in *your* life right now? I thought so. Something tells me it didn't take you very long, because when you're still angry or upset with somebody for something they did a while back, it takes a while for those feelings to go away. But for every minute you spend thinking about somebody who did you wrong, that's another minute you could've been thinking optimistically and moving your life in a healthier direction.

Now look, I'm not saying to forgive somebody who really did something horrible to you or someone close to you (or to anyone, for that matter). And I'm not saying to bring this person back into your life, especially if there's the potential of them still being a negative influence on you.

Instead, I want you to give some serious thought to anyone in your life who may have fallen out of favor, check that list with those closest to you (for a better perspective on whether you might be holding a grudge longer than you should be), then reach out to that person and forgive them. What you'll get back might not be an apology, but what you'll have is peace of mind that you tried, as well as more time to think about positive thoughts instead of negative ones.

STRIVE to talk instead of type. I'm entirely guilty of texting instead of calling people when things are hectic and I feel like I'm in the middle of trying to get a million things done. I mean, come on. It's too easy to stay connected with people through texts, emails, and posts, but that's just it—it's **too** easy, which is the whole point.

The fact that typing to somebody instead of talking to them *is* so easy and convenient is what also makes anything we type less meaningful. Am I saying to never text your friends? Yeah, no— that would be both insane and impossible. But own the fact that every time you choose typing instead of talking, you're giving someone you supposedly care about a little bit less of yourself.

Even though you can stay connected that way, you're accepting the fact that you don't need to communicate with them on a deeper level. That you would rather see an LOL on a screen instead of hearing them crack up over the phone, or better yet, in person. That your friendship can easily grow without putting more than a handful of minutes into it.

That said, typing something out may be necessary sometimes, but face it, it's not necessary *all* the time—and the less you do it, the stronger the bonds you'll have with the people you're speaking to more often. And if you don't believe that, just ask yourself: If I called you instead with the advice I just shared, would my words have more meaning hearing me *say* them as opposed to you *reading* them? If the answer's yes, then never doubt that whoever you're calling feels the same way about yours.

STRIVE to help others strive. When I find something I absolutely love to do that moves me, I don't just go at it crazy hard. I want to share it with others, especially if it's something I feel others could benefit from too.

That's how this book got started. Just by talking about my approach to life after Sjögren's and how STRIVING had helped me through it made others around me eager to try it. By sharing it with them, I actually found it easier to STRIVE, because now, I'm not alone doing it. Little by little, I found myself surrounded by a few friends and family making the same promises to themselves to STRIVE every day. That's why I encourage you to talk about this process with anybody who's curious about what's going on with you.

Would I love them to join the ranks and do it with you? Please, that's a no-brainer. But even if they're not curious to try it, by explaining STRIVE to them, you'll give those around you a better understanding of what you're doing for yourself and how you're trying to improve your life. That alone will keep you from having to explain your actions or choices as often, earn their support, and who knows—maybe convince them down the road to give it a try for themselves. Because if you really care about them, wouldn't you want them to have the best life possible too?

STRIVE—With Yourself

Like I said at the beginning of this chapter, there's always more room to grow. Wherever you start is not where you have to end—and wherever you are right now doesn't have to be your last step forward.

Life is all about change, and you don't have to do one thing forever—believe me, I know. You should always be moving forward, and once you finally realize one goal—no matter how great or how small it was—it's important to immediately have a new one in place. The very definition of the word *strive* is to reach for something above and beyond, so the only true way to continue to STRIVE is by reaching for something else that's just out of reach after you've grasped your last goal.

But I don't want you to think that you have to take some huge risk and change everything about yourself or your life. For example, a lot of people think that entrepreneurs take big risks, as if they're dropping everything they love and quitting school for their dream. Maybe a handful went that way, but most entrepreneurs still work their day jobs while trying to start a business. Sure, they take risks, but at the same time, those risks are tempered. Look at the life of Madam C. J. Walker, America's very first female Black self-made millionaire. She literally created her cosmetics and hair-care line for Black women *while* still working as a sales agent. Instead of quitting her day job, she kept selling as an entrepreneur-philanthropist while she built her side hustle into a successful business that would eventually train nearly twenty thousand to become sales agents for her business.

Personally, I'm now at the point where I finally realize that I can't say yes to everything anymore because that often prevents me from doing my best with whatever it is that I'm doing. Because of that, I've gotten quite picky about what I STRIVE to do, and that is exactly where I want you to be.

STRIVING is about taking that next step—having that next goal for yourself—and there are so many ways to move yourself forward that the ones I'll mention here only scratch the surface. So, think about what you want for yourself—what that next goal is—but make sure that what you choose is enough of a change to make a difference but not so difficult that it negatively affects any other parts of your life you've already improved on.

STRIVE to conquer the five. What "five" am I talking about? I mean the five conditions that lead to metabolic syndrome (also called insulin resistance syndrome):

1. **A large waistline:** A waist circumference of thirty-five inches or more (women) or forty-plus inches (men).
2. **High blood pressure:** Anything over 130/85.
3. **High blood sugar:** Glucose levels above one hundred mg/dL.
4. **Low levels of good cholesterol (HDL):** Lower than fifty mg/dL (in women) or lower than forty mg/dL (in men); or needing to take medication to keep it under control.
5. **High triglyceride levels:** Higher than 150 mg/dL, or requiring medication to manage it.

Having just three or more of these conditions (on a consistent basis) significantly raises your risk of diabetes, stroke, coronary heart disease, and other serious health-related problems, such as cancer, bone loss, brain health issues, kidney and nerve damage, and even dementia. The bad news is roughly one in three adults has metabolic syndrome in the United States. The good news is, by trying many of the techniques in this book, you'll already be on the way to changing these five in your favor.

Now, obviously, these take time to address, as well as certain equipment (like a blood pressure monitor and a tape measure), blood tests (which your doctor could provide), and quite honestly, a little patience, depending on where you are presently. But when you keep these five under control, it puts you in the driver's seat of your own health in a way that may literally save your life—now that's something to STRIVE for!

STRIVE by overcoming a fear. I'm not talking about swimming with sharks, jumping out of an airplane, or anything crazy like that. In fact, I want you to start with something entirely safe and harmless, but for some reason, makes you anxious, scared, or uncomfortable. It doesn't have to be just trying something new or petrifying, BTW. For example, trying something that's not scary whatsoever but that you're afraid to fail at also counts.

Whatever fear you decide to overcome doesn't have to be healthy. I mean, volunteering to do improv in front of a bunch of total strangers might get your heart rate up, but I wouldn't call it aerobic exercise. It could be an activity you're afraid you'll look foolish doing, trying a food that's healthy but disgusting, talking to a particular person who makes you nervous, anything that—if given the choice—you'd be entirely fine with never trying for the rest of your life.

Why would I want you to put yourself through that torture? Well, to prove to yourself that you can do what you set out to do, even if it's something you absolutely don't want to. Because when you STRIVE in this direction and succeed, you create an example that you're capable of more than you might give yourself credit for, and that example can go a long way in getting you to repeat that courage repeatedly with other things.

You see, the choices you make to stay fit, eat right, maintain healthy relationships, and stay true to yourself are yours to make— but often, we choose what we're most comfortable with. But with so many other smart choices out there, knowing that you can overcome anything will give you the confidence to walk toward, not away from, the next healthy opportunity that comes your way.

Finally—STRIVE to try something not in this book. Does this book contain every possible way you could **STRIVE** with your life? Of course not, just as it doesn't list everything you technically could **observe, appreciate, balance, enrich, soothe, believe,** and **inspire**. But what book could ever do that without being the size of an encyclopedia set? And how boring would it be if the only things you could ever improve about your life were that limited?

So, let me ask you a couple of questions:

- Was there anything you didn't find in this book that you expected to see suggested?
- Was there anything I briefly touched on that you're now more curious about?

If the answer is yes to either, then that's awesome, because that's what I wanted to hear. I want you thinking about how you could add to STRIVE, because like I said upfront, the advice in this book is just a variety of approaches you could try. But the real key to a better life is following the road map of **observing**, **appreciating**, **balancing**, **enriching**, **soothing**, **believing**, **inspiring**, and **STRIVING** every single day from this day forward.

So, what are you going to add to the formula? What new and exciting food choices, activities, techniques, and philosophies did I leave out that you want to put in? It's up to you, but promise me this. Whatever you choose to bring to STRIVE, make sure that it lets you keep the same promise to yourself that I made to myself:

Make it easy, make it enjoyable,
but—most of all—make it exciting.

CHAPTER 11

THE STRIVE STRATEGY

The magic of STRIVE is that it's all about remembering the eight actions and applying them as often as possible to the four major areas of your life.

Now, do I expect you to **observe, appreciate, balance, enrich, soothe, believe, inspire,** and **STRIVE** in all four major areas of your life—your **diet**, your **activities, who and what's around you,** and **yourself**—every single day?

Are you kidding me? Please. I know I've never pulled that off myself—not once—and this is *my* personal philosophy. Besides, trying to do all that in one day would only stress me out and completely break that promise I made to myself. I don't think anyone would find it easy, enjoyable, or exciting trying to do thirty-two things a day, do you?

But then again—maybe you would.

That's why this program allows a lot of flexibility. Each day, you get to choose how you want to STRIVE. As you'll start to figure out, the combinations may be endless, but you can always depend on seeing amazing results!

Short STRIVING

Remember what I said at the beginning of the book? That you were a success if, before you went to sleep, you can say to yourself:

- I **observed** something today.
- I **appreciated** something today.
- I **balanced** something today.
- I **enriched** something today.
- I **soothed** something today.
- I **believed** in something today.
- I **inspired** someone today—either myself or someone else.
- I **strove** toward something today.

That's what I call *Short STRIVING*. You can pick and choose which areas of your life you want to make an impact on that day. For example, you might choose to **observe**, **balance**, and **believe** in your *diet*, **appreciate**, and **STRIVE** in your *activities*, **enrich**, **soothe**, and **inspire** *who and what's around you*—and never get around to focusing on *yourself*. So long as you completed all eight actions for the day, you're STRIVING! Mix and match as you please!

It's the bare minimum, but that doesn't make it any less effective than any of the other suggestions you'll soon read about. In fact, it's a great starting place to help you get the hang of STRIVE before you really begin exploring the program's possibilities.

It's also a great way to STRIVE on days when you might not have as much time, so don't be afraid to use it, even if you consider yourself advanced and have been STRIVING for a while.

Strict STRIVING

nstead of randomly jumping around between **diet, activities, who and what's around you**, and **yourself**—try focusing all eight actions on **just one** of those areas for the day.

For example: if you decide to Strict STRIVE your activities to-day, then you'll do at least one thing to **observe, appreciate, balance, enrich, soothe, believe, inspire**, and **STRIVE** with your *activities* that day. No doing *just* seven of the eight actions and skipping one. It's about jumping in with both feet and putting all your attention on STRIVING just in that area of your life that day—no exceptions.

Can you Strict STRIVE for more than one area of your life on the same day? Meaning, could you have a day where you focus on your diet and yourself at the same time? Your activities and who and what's around you at the same time—doing all eight actions for both? Sure. I won't stop you from attempting to focus on more than one area on the same day if you think you can. Just remember—so long as it still feels easy, enjoyable, and exciting, then you're good.

Serious STRIVING

f you're up for a challenge, this is it. Serious STRIVING is about checking off every single box in all four areas of your life—all in the same day. That means I expect you to **observe, appreciate, balance, enrich, soothe, believe, inspire**, and **STRIVE** with your *diet, your activities, who and what's around you*, and *yourself* throughout the course of the day. Do the math and that's tech-nically thirty-two things you're accountable for. That's a lot, but remember, it's why I call it Serious STRIVING. If it was any easier, I'd have to think of another title for it.

If you go through the book, you'll find there are ways you can sort of "check off the boxes" with less effort than it sounds like, using easier tricks and tactics so that doing thirty-two tasks in one day isn't as overwhelming. Not that I'm suggesting you take the easy road. I'm just saying that, yes, it's a challenge—but it can be a lot more doable than you think. Just keep this in mind if you attempt it:

If you fail, you're still a winner: What if, by the end of the night, you never managed to do all thirty-two? Maybe you hit fifteen, twenty, or worse—pulled off thirty-one and just missed it by one. Well, guess what? That's thirty-one healthy things you did for yourself today that you wouldn't have done otherwise. That's not losing—that's succeeding, even if you were lucky to do half of what you had planned on.

If you're desperate, then dial it back: Meaning, if you're attempting a Serious STRIVE because you just want to see results as quickly as possible, please don't do it. Trying to go from zero to one hundred miles per hour before you're ready to, just because you want to make your life better instantaneously, isn't the right mindset to be in.

Like I said, even a Short STRIVE will improve your life because you're doing things for yourself you never did before or never did as often as you should have. This is your *life* we're talking about, so don't rush through things because you can't wait. The results will come—you must trust the process.

STRIVE Q & A

"Can I repeat the exact same tasks the next day?"

Theoretically, sure. I mean, you're still doing eight positive things for yourself that next day. And you might be so satisfied with how today went that you may think, "Why mess with a good thing?" and want to repeat that same magic tomorrow, right? As long as you still enjoy what you're doing, that's what counts.

However, what you'll start to discover is that the more you repeat certain positive things, the quicker and more likely many of them will become a healthy habit. Suddenly, instead of having to think about balancing your meals, you'll find you do it without giving it a thought. Instead of thinking about having to stretch, it just becomes part of your day because you enjoy it.

My point being, if anything becomes second nature to you and eventually becomes part of your daily routine, keep that positive habit in play but consider trying something different to give yourself credit so you grow even further.

"What should I do once I reach one of my goals?"

Everybody's definition of living the best life possible is different. Maybe in your case, you're turning to STRIVE to try and lose a few pounds before vacation? Boost your energy to keep up with your kids? Lower your cholesterol because your doctor told you to? All the above?

No matter what you were hoping to improve, once you've achieved that goal, the first thing to do is celebrate yourself. You did it! I may have showed you a different path than you've tried before to reach your goal, but you're the one who stayed on that path and got there. And if you stay on the path, that goal is forever in your reach.

But after that, I want you to consider this: If even **STRIVE** was a means to a certain end for you, that doesn't mean your journey is over. This isn't about just about improving a certain portion of yourself—STRIVE is about improving your entire life for the better. The longer you stick with it—even if you've achieved what you were initially hoping to change—the more positive changes you'll make and the closer you'll be toward an even better version of yourself.

"Can I just skip one of the actions?"

Trust me when I say that all eight actions deserve your equal respect. They're all intertwined and build upon each other, affecting one another both directly and indirectly in the smallest to most impactful ways. But when you don't address all eight, it can make things a lot harder to stay dedicated to a healthy lifestyle.

Even if you can't see some of those connections now, you're going to start noticing them the more you STRIVE. And as you begin to adopt more healthier habits in one area of your life, it will start making other habits in other areas of your life not only easier to do but more likely to show results as well. It all depends on where your life is now and where the eight actions take you.

"Okay, but what happens if I don't do all eight actions?"

Hey, life gets in the way sometimes, and it's entirely understandable that, occasionally, you might end the day realizing you didn't pull off all eight. In fact, I expect it'll happen, especially early in the program as you start to adopt the mindset. But when it does, be proud of yourself for the actions you managed to pull off that day, then ask yourself the following questions:

How much effort did I put in? If you gave it your all, then we're good. But if you didn't—and only you know the answer to that—then accept that you could've tried harder. Then try harder tomorrow. Remember—you can do this.

Did anyone or anything stand in the way? Maybe someone or something was the reason you couldn't pull off all eight actions. If so, think about how you might be able to prevent that from happening the next time.

Did I try them in the wrong order? Some actions might be easier for you at certain times of the day, while others might be more difficult. Give some thought to *when* you might've tried an action you couldn't complete, then rearrange them accordingly to work in your favor.

Did I bite off more than I could chew? Maybe the reason you didn't finish an action was because it was too hard for you, not just that day, but because it was just too much to tackle. If that's the case, dial it back a bit and find a different task to try the next time. Get a few days where you're able to pull off all eight actions, then maybe come back to it with a little more confidence and experience.

Finally, do I care that I couldn't complete all eight? Weird question, right? Here's the thing though—you should. Because if you don't, then you're not invested in this enough to make huge strides with your life.

Remember, if you allow yourself to slide today without wishing you had done better, it only makes it a little easier to let yourself slide tomorrow. That's a slippery slope I don't want you to ever get on. If you want your life to change, you should feel some regret but not enough that you beat yourself up. But it's critical that you care about doing your best, because that's the only way you'll see the greatest results possible.

And that's it!

Look, what I've shared are just a handful of ways you can use the program. Can you get creative on your own and think of other ways to STRIVE that are different from what I'm suggesting? Are there additional choices you could make to eat better, different exercises you could try to get in shape, or other ways to make a positive impact on your overall health? Are there other things you could be observing, appreciating, balancing, and so on with your life? The answer is 100 percent yes.

STRIVE is just a guide—a variety of ideas and methods you could apply to make a difference in your life. But that doesn't mean you have to use all of them to succeed—and it doesn't mean you can't bring a few of your own to the table.

STRIVE is a jumping-off point for you to start but definitely not where you should stop. Like I mentioned at the end of Chapter 10, the final thing to STRIVE for is figuring out even more ways to STRIVE so that the program grows alongside you. Because of that adaptability, even though I personally can't wait to see how this program transforms you—I'm even more excited about where you end up taking the program.

Happy STRIVING!

ACKNOWLEDGMENTS

I have always believed that as long as the sun comes up, you have a chance. A chance to live your dreams. A chance for a first chance or a second chance. A chance to go for it, fail or succeed, and go for it again! That chance and the ability to STRIVE first starts with the gift of life. It is such a blessing to have this overwhelmingly beautiful and undeserved gift of life, and I thank my God Jehovah for this blessing.

The writing of this book was a team effort, and none of this could have been achieved without the vision of Mel Berger. Thank you for your continued belief in me and your direction in this effort. You are a legend!

Myatt Murphy was and is a true hero in championing this book and capturing my voice in each word we crafted together. We make the perfect doubles team! You truly get me and enhanced even my vision for this book. This effort would have been impossible without you. Your concept of what it means to STRIVE could only be understood by a fellow striver. Your ability to capture what it means to strive is truly genius.

As of the date of publishing this book, my agent of twenty-five years, Carlos Fleming, has overseen my on-court and off-court exploits. The vision for telling my story is coming to life and I can't wait for the next steps in this journey of written word. I can't wait for these coming years to unfold to show you all what we have planned!

Striving all starts with having a strong set of values, and that often comes with having a strong set of role models. My mom and dad couldn't be more perfect in that regard. I want to be just like you. No one's strides are longer than you both.

Many times the best teachers are those who show you with their actions without saying a word. My sisters Isha and Lyndrea both personify that in all ways. Thank you for taking the lead and setting a good example for me both in how you live your lives and setting a good example for me spiritually. I know you would do anything for me and it makes me feel so special, safe, and happy to know that I always have you there.

I will never be just Venus, it's always Venus and Serena. So many of my stories and experiences come from learning from my little sister. You are the most courageous and fearless person I know. I've learned so much from you, Serena, and I continue to learn from you now as a wife and a mom. Thank you for showing me how to be a champion

A special thanks to my friend Lara Shriftman, who took it upon herself to make sure this book was in everyone's hands. You always go above and beyond for those you love, and it's so wonderful to be counted as one of your loved ones.

A special thank you to those in my life who mean so much to me. Sonya Haffey who I have the most respect and admiration for. You embody what a truly good human being is. Thank you for sharing your talent and time with me all these years.

To all my nieces and nephews, Jeffery, Justus, Jair, Olympia, Adira, and Amir, you all are the joys of my life. My biggest dream is for you to strive and dream for all desire. This book is for you.

And finally, but not least, to all the readers. It gives me so much joy seeing people thrive, be genuinely well, and lead happy, fulfilling lives. Building a good life is like playing a match. You practice, you prepare, and you develop the techniques for success until executing them becomes easy and second nature. Striving is a technique for life. How to practice a successful life involves training and intention, but doesn't have to be hard and should be joyful, especially as you see it work in your life. It pains me to see people hurt and sad based on the situations they put themselves in. Whether through lack of values, lack of confidence, or other reasons, it's my hope that striving can help each reader toward an easier path to happiness and success through an examination of self and everyday habits. Happy Striving!

Chapter 5: Balance

1. Diane S. Lauderdale et al., "Sleep Duration: How Well Do Self-Reports Reflect Objective Measures? The CARDIA Sleep Study," *Epidemiology* 19, no. 6 (November 2008): 838–45.

Chapter 6: Enrich

1. S. K. Verma, Vartika Jain, and S. S. Katewa, "Blood Pressure Lowering, Fibrinolysis Enhancing and Antioxidant Activities of Cardamom (*Elettaria Cardamomum*)," *Indian Journal of Biochemistry & Biophysics* 46, no. 6 (December 2009): 503–6.

2. Vijayalakshmi Prabhakaran, Thenmozhi Sengodan, and Palaniappan Rajeswari, "The Evaluation of the Virulence Factors of Clinical *Candida* Isolates and the Anti-biofilm Activity of *Elettaria cardamomum* against Multi-drug Resistant *Candida albicans*," *Current Medical Mycology* 2, no. 2 (June 2016): 8–15.

3. Mark F. McCarty, James DiNicolantonio, and James O'Keefe, "Capsaicin May Have Important Potential for Promoting Vascular and Metabolic Health," *Open Heart* 2, no. 1 (June 2015): e000262, https://doi .org/10.1136/openhrt-2015-000262.

4. P. Ranasinghe et al., "Efficacy and Safety of 'True' Cinnamon (*Cinnamomum zeylanicum*) as a Pharmaceutical Agent in Diabetes: A Systematic Review and Meta-Analysis," *Diabetic Medicine* 29 (June 2012): 1480–92, https://doi.org/10.1111/j.1464-5491.2012.03718.x.

5. Shatadal Ghosh, Sharmistha Banerjee, and Parames Sil, "The Beneficial Role of Curcumin on Inflammation, Diabetes, and Neurodegenerative Disease: A Recent Update," *Food and Chemical Toxicology* 83, no. 6 (September 2015): 111–24, https://doi.org/10.1016/j.fct.2015.05.022.

6. Pietro Dulbecco and Vincenzo Savarino, "Therapeutic Potential of Cur-

cumin in Digestive Diseases," *The World Journal of Gastroenterology* 19, no. 48 (December 2013): 9256–70, https://doi.org/10.3748/wjg.v19 .i48.9256.

7. Jayaraj Ravindran, Sahdeo Prasad, and Bharat B. Aggarwal, "Curcumin and Cancer Cells: How Many Ways Can Curry Kill Tumor Cells Selectively?," *The AAPS Journal* 11, no. 3: 495–510, https://doi.org/10.1208 /s12248-009-9128-x.

8. Edzard Ernst and M. H. Pittler, "Efficacy of Ginger for Nausea and Vomiting: A Systematic Review of Randomized Clinical Trials," *British Journal of Anaesthesia* 84, no. 3 (March 2000): 367–71.

9. Nafiseh Shokri-Mashhadi et al., "Anti-Oxidative and Anti-Inflammatory Effects of Ginger in Health and Physical Activity: Review of Current Evidence," Supplement, *International Journal of Preventative Medicine* 4, no. S1 (April 2013): S36–S42.

10. Isabella Savini et al., "Origanum Vulgare Induces Apoptosis in Human Colon Cancer Caco2 Cells," *Nutrition and Cancer* 61, no. 3 (2009): 381–89; Bonn University, "Salutary Pizza Spice: Oregano Helps against Inflammations," *ScienceDaily* (June 2008), www.sciencedaily.com/releases /2008/06/080625093147.htm.

11. Nayely Leyva-López et al., "Essential Oils of Oregano: Biological Activity beyond Their Antimicrobial Properties," *Molecules* 22, no. 6 (June 2017): 989, https://doi.org/10.3390/molecules22060989.

12. A. N. Panche, A. D. Diwan, and S. R. Chandra, "Flavonoids: An Overview," *Journal of Nutritional Science* 5 (December 2016): e47, https://doi .org/10.1017/jns.2016.41.

13. Jessy Moore, Michael Yousef, and Evangelia Tsiani, "Anticancer Effects of Rosemary (*Rosmarinus officinalis* L.) Extract and Rosemary Extract Polyphenols," *Nutrients* 8, no. 11 (November 2016): 731.

14. Monika Sienkiewicz et al., "The Potential of Use Basil and Rosemary Essential Oils as Effective Antibacterial Agents," *Molecules* 18, no. 8 (August 2013): 9334–51.

15. Bahare Salehi et al., "Thymol, Thyme, and Other Plant Sources: Health and Potential Uses," *Phytotherapy Research* 32, no. 9 (September 2018): 1688–1706.

16. Bharat B. Aggarwal, "Targeting Inflammation-Induced Obesity and Metabolic Diseases by Curcumin and Other Nutraceuticals," *Annual Review Nutrition* 30, (2010): 173–99, https://doi.org/10.1146/annurev.nutr .012809.104755.

17. University of Illinois at Urbana-Champaign, "Dark Honey Has More

Illness-Fighting Agents Than Light Honey," ScienceDaily (July 1998), https://www.sciencedaily.com/releases/1998/07/980708085352.htm.

18. Sung-Chuan Chao et al., "Induction of Sirtuin-1 Signaling by Resveratrol Induces Human Chondrosarcoma Cell Apoptosis and Exhibits Antitumor Activity," *Scientific Reports* 9, no. 1 (June 2017): 3180, https://doi.org/10.1038/s41598-017-03635-7.

Chapter 7: Soothe

1. Qingyi Huang et al., "Linking What We Eat to Our Mood: A Review of Diet, Dietary Antioxidants, and Depression," *Antioxidants* 8, no. 9 (September 2019): 376, https://doi.org/10.3390/antiox8090376.

2. Glenda Lindseth, Brian Helland, and Julie Caspers, "The Effects of Dietary Tryptophan on Affective Disorders," *Archives of Psychiatric Nursing* 29, no. 2 (December 2014): 102–7, https://doi.org/10.1016/j.apnu.2014.11.008.

Chapter 8: Believe

1. Andrew Reynolds et al., "Carbohydrate Quality and Human Health: A Series of Systematic Reviews and Meta-Analyses," *Lancet* 393, no. 10170 (January 2019): 434–45, https://doi.org/10.1016/S0140-6736(18)31809-9.

2. Andrea Bellavia et al., "Fruit and Vegetable Consumption and All-Cause Mortality: A Dose-Response Analysis," *The American Journal of Clinical Nutrition* 98, no. 2 (June 2013): 454–59, https://doi.org/10.3945/ajcn.112.056119.

3. Yuan-Ting Lo et al., "Spending on Vegetable and Fruit Consumption Could Reduce All-Cause Mortality among Older Adults," *Nutrition Journal* 11, (December 2012): 113, https://doi.org/10.1186/1475-2891-11-113.

4. National Center for Health Statistics, "Obesity and Overweight," Centers for Disease Control and Prevention, January 5, 2023, https://www.cdc.gov/nchs/fastats/obesity-overweight.htm.

5. Ian Janssen et al., "Years of Life Gained Due to Leisure-Time Physical Activity in the US," *American Journal of Preventive Medicine* 44, no. 1 (January 2013): 23–29, https://doi.org/10.1016/j.amepre.2012.09.056.

6. Mayo Clinic Staff, "Aerobic Exercise: Top 10 Reasons to Get Physical," Mayo Clinic, http://www.mayoclinic.com/health/aerobic-exercise/EP00002/NSECTIONGROUP=2.

7. James W. Anderson, Chunxu Liu, and Richard J. Kryscio, "Blood Pressure Response to Transcendental Meditation: A Meta-Analysis," *Ameri-*

can Journal of Hypertension 21, no. 3 (January 2008): 310–16, https://doi
.org/10.1038/ajh.2007.65.

8. Márcia de Fátima Rosas Marchiori et al., "Decrease in Blood Pressure
    and Improved Psychological Aspects through Meditation Training in
    Hypertensive Older Adults: A Randomized Control Study," *Geriatrics
    and Gerontology International* 15, no. 10 (November 2014): 1158–64,
    https://doi.org/10.1111/ggi.12414.

9. Jason C. Ong et al., "A Randomized Controlled Trial of Mindfulness
    Meditation for Chronic Insomnia," *Sleep* 37, no. 9 (September 2014):
    1553–63, https://doi.org/10.5665/sleep.4010.

10. Tonya L. Jacobs et al., "Intensive Meditation Training, Immune Cell
    Telomerase Activity, and Psychological Mediators," *Psychoneuroendocri-
    nology* 36, no. 5 (June 2011): 664–81, https://doi.org/10.1016/j.psyneuen
    .2010.09.010.

11. Amit Mohan, Ratna Sharma, and Ramesh L. Bijlani, "Effect of Medita-
    tion on Stress-Induced Changes in Cognitive Functions," *The Journal of
    Alternative and Complementary Medicine* 17, no. 3 (March 2011): 207–
    12, https://doi.org/10.1089/acm.2010.0142.

12. Andrew B. Newberg et al., "Meditation Effects on Cognitive Function
    and Cerebral Blood Flow in Subjects with Memory Loss: A Preliminary
    Study," *Journal of Alzheimer's Disease* 20, no. 2 (2010): 517–26, https://
    doi.org/10.3233/JAD-2010-1391.

13. Yi-Yuan Tang et al., "Mechanisms of White Matter Changes Induced
    by Meditation," *Proceedings of the National Academy of Sciences of the
    United States of America* 109, no. 26 (June 2012): 10570–74, https://doi
    .org/10.1073/pnas.1207817109.

14. Manoj K. Bhasin et al., "Relaxation Response Induces Temporal Tran-
    scriptome Changes in Energy Metabolism, Insulin Secretion, and In-
    flammatory Pathways," *PLoS One* 8, no. 5 (May 2013): e62817, https://
    doi.org/10.1371/journal.pone.0062817.

15. Shawn N. Katterman et al., "Mindfulness Meditation as an Interven-
    tion for Binge Eating, Emotional Eating, and Weight Loss: A Systematic
    Review," *Eating Behaviors* 15, no. 2 (April 2014): 197–204, https://doi
    .org/10.1016/j.eatbeh.2014.01.005.

16. Peter la Cour and Marian Petersen, "Effects of Mindfulness Meditation
    on Chronic Pain: A Randomized Controlled Trial," *Pain Medicine* 14, no.
    4 (April 2015): 641–52, https://doi.org/10.1111/pme.12605.

17. Debra Umberson and Jennifer Karas Montez, "Social Relationships
    and Health: A Flashpoint for Health Policy," Supplement, *Journal of*

Health Social Behavior 51, no. S1 (2010): S54–S66, https://doi.org/10
.1177/0022146510383501.

18. Sakda Hewagalamulage et al., "Stress, Cortisol, and Obesity: A Role for Cortisol Responsiveness in Identifying Individuals Prone to Obesity," Supplement, *Domestic Animal Endocrinology* 56, (July 2016): S112–20, https://doi.org/10.1016/j.domaniend.2016.03.004.

19. Rachel K. Narr et al., "Close Friendship Strength and Broader Peer Group Desirability as Differential Predictors of Adult Mental Health," *Child Development* 90, no. 1 (January 2019): 298–313, https://doi.org/10.1111/cdev.12905.

20. Michael L. M. Murphy, Denise Janicki-Deverts, and Sheldon Cohen, "Receiving a Hug Is Associated with the Attenuation of Negative Mood that Occurs on Days with Interpersonal Conflict," *PLoS One* 13, no. 10 (October 2018): e0203522, https://doi.org/10.1371/journal.pone.0203522.

21. Kimberley J. Smith et al., "The Association between Loneliness, Social Isolation and Inflammation: A Systematic Review and Meta-Analysis," *Neuroscience & Biobehavioral Reviews* 112, (February 2020): 519–41, https://doi.org/10.1016/j.neubiorev.2020.02.002.

22. Amanda Cook Maher et al., "Psychological Well-Being in Elderly Adults with Extraordinary Episodic Memory," *PLoS One* 12, no. 10 (October 2017): e0186413, https://doi.org/10.1371/journal.pone.0186413.

23. Rosemary Blieszner, Aaron M. Ogletree, and Rebecca G. Adams, "Friendship in Later Life: A Research Agenda," *Innovation in Aging* 3, no. 1 (March 2019): igz005, https://doi.org/10.1093/geroni/igz005.

24. Pavel Goldstein, Irit Weissman-Fogel, and Simone G. Shamay-Tsoory, "The Role of Touch in Regulating Inter-Partner Physiological Coupling during Empathy for Pain," *Scientific Reports* 7, no. 1 (June 2017): 3252, https://doi.org/10.1038/s41598-017-03627-7.

25. Joel Salinas et al., "Association of Social Support with Brain Volume and Cognition," *JAMA Network Open* 4, no. 8 (2021): e2121122, https://doi.org/10.1001/jamanetworkopen.2021.21122.

26. Julianne Holt-Lunstad, Timothy B. Smith, and J. Bradley Layton, "Social Relationships and Mortality Risk: A Meta-Analytic Review," *PLoS Medicine* 7, no. 7 (July 2010): e1000316, https://doi.org/10.1371/journal.pmed.1000316.

27. Xiaolin Xu et al., "Social Relationship Satisfaction and Accumulation of Chronic Conditions and Multimorbidity: A National Cohort of Australian Women," *General Psychiatry* 36, no. 1 (February 2023): e100925, https://doi.org/10.1136/gpsych-2022-100925.

Chapter 9: Inspire

1. Caoimhe Twohig-Bennett and Andy Jones, "The Health Benefits of the Great Outdoors: A Systematic Review and Meta-Analysis of Greenspace Exposure and Health Outcomes," *Environmental Research* 166 (October 2018): 628–37, https://doi.org/10.1016/j.envres.2018.06.030.

Chapter 10: STRIVE

1. Carmen Sayon-Orea et al., "Reported Fried Food Consumption and the Incidence of Hypertension in a Mediterranean Cohort: The SUN (Seguimiento Universidad de Navarra) Project," *British Journal of Nutrition* 112, no. 6 (September 2014): 984–91, https://doi.org/10.1017/S0007114514001755.
2. Leah E. Cahill et al., "Fried-Food Consumption and Risk of Type 2 Diabetes and Coronary Artery Disease: A Prospective Study in 2 Cohorts of US Women and Men," *The American Journal of Clinical Nutrition* 100, no. 2 (August 2014): 667–75, https://doi.org/10.3945/ajcn.114.084129.

Aggarwal, Bharat B. "Targeting Inflammation-Induced Obesity and Metabolic Diseases by Curcumin and Other Nutraceuticals." *Annual Review Nutrition* 30 (2010): 173–99. https://doi.org/10.1146/annurev.nutr.012809.104755.

Anderson, James W., Chunxu Liu, and Richard J. Kryscio. "Blood Pressure Response to Transcendental Meditation: A Meta-Analysis." *American Journal of Hypertension* 21, no. 3 (January 2008): 310–16. https://doi.org/10.1038/ajh.2007.65.

Bellavia, Andrea, Susanna C. Larsson, Matteo Bottai, Alicja Wolk, and Nicola Orsini. "Fruit and Vegetable Consumption and All-Cause Mortality: A Dose-Response Analysis." *The American Journal of Clinical Nutrition* 98, no. 2 (June 2013): 454–59. https://doi.org/10.3945/ajcn.112.056119.

Bhasin, Manoj K., Jeffery A. Dusek, Bei-Hung Chang, Marie G. Joseph, John W. Denninger, Gregory L. Fricchione, Herbert Benson, and Towia A. Libermann. "Relaxation Response Induces Temporal Transcriptome Changes in Energy Metabolism, Insulin Secretion, and Inflammatory Pathways." *PLoS One* 8, no. 5 (May 2013): e62817. https://doi.org/10.1371/journal.pone.0062817.

Blieszner, Rosemary, Aaron M. Ogletree, and Rebecca G. Adams. "Friendship in Later Life: A Research Agenda." *Innovation in Aging* 3, no. 1 (March 2019): igz005. https://doi.org/10.1093/geroni/igz005.

Bonn University. "Salutary Pizza Spice: Oregano Helps Against Inflammations." *ScienceDaily* (June 2008). www.sciencedaily.com/releases/2008/06/080625093147.htm.

Cahill, Leah E., An Pan, Stephanie E. Chiuve, Qi Sun, Walter C. Willett, Frank B. Hu, and Eric B. Rimm. "Fried-Food Consumption and Risk of Type 2 Diabetes and Coronary Artery Disease: A Prospective Study in 2 Cohorts of US Women and Men." *The American Journal of Clinical Nutrition* 100, no. 2 (August 2014): 667–75. https://doi.org/10.3945/ajcn.114.084129.

Chao, Sung-Chuan, Ying-Ju Chen, Kuo-How Huang, Kuan-Lin Kuo, Ting-Hua Yang, Kuo-Yuan Huang, Ching-Chia Wang, Chih-Hsin Tang, Rong-Sen Yang, and Shing-Hwa Liu. "Induction of Sirtuin-1 Signaling by Resveratrol Induces Human Chondrosarcoma Cell Apoptosis and Exhibits Antitumor Activity." *Scientific Reports* 9, no. 1 (June 2017): 3180. https://doi.org/10.1038/s41598-017-03635-7.

Cook Maher, Amanda, Stephanie Kielb, Emmaleigh Loyer, Maureen Connelley, Alfred Rademaker, M.-Marsel Mesulam, Sandra Weintraub, Dan McAdams, Regina Logan, and Emily Rogalski. "Psychological Well-Being in Elderly Adults with Extraordinary Episodic Memory." *PLoS One* 12, no. 10 (October 2017): e0186413. https://doi.org/10.1371/journal.pone.0186413.

de Fátima Rosas Marchiori, Márcia, Elisa Kozasa, Roberto Dischinger Miranda, André Luiz Monezi Andrade, Tatiana Caccese Perrotti, and José Roberto Leite. "Decrease in Blood Pressure and Improved Psychological Aspects through Meditation Training in Hypertensive Older Adults: A Randomized Control Study." *Geriatrics and Gerontology International* 15, no. 10 (November 2014): 1158–64. https://doi.org/10.1111/ggi.12414.

Dulbecco, Pietro, and Vincenzo Savarino. "Therapeutic Potential of Curcumin in Digestive Diseases." *The World Journal of Gastroenterology* 19, no. 48 (December 2013): 9256–70. https://doi.org/10.3748/wjg.v19.i48.9256.

Ernst, Edzard, and M. H. Pittler. "Efficacy of Ginger for Nausea and Vomiting: A Systematic Review of Randomized Clinical Trials." *British Journal of Anaesthesia* 84, no. 3 (March 2000): 367–71.

Ghosh, Shatadal, Sharmistha Banerjee, and Parames Sil. "The Beneficial Role of Curcumin on Inflammation, Diabetes, and Neurodegenerative Disease: A Recent Update." *Food and Chemical Toxicology* 83, no. 6 (September 2015): 111–24. https://doi.org/10.1016/j.fct.2015.05.022.

Goldstein, Pavel, Irit Weissman-Fogel, and Simone G. Shamay-Tsoory. "The Role of Touch in Regulating Inter-Partner Physiological Coupling during Empathy for Pain." *Scientific Reports* 7, no. 1 (June 2017): 3252. https://doi.org/10.1038/s41598-017-03627-7.

Hewagalamulage, Sakda, T. Kevin Lee, Iain J. Clarke, and Belinda Henry. "Stress, Cortisol, and Obesity: A Role for Cortisol Responsiveness in Identifying Individuals Prone to Obesity." Supplement, *Domestic Animal Endocrinology* 56, (July 2016): S112–20. https://doi.org/10.1016/j.domaniend.2016.03.004.

Holt-Lunstad, Julianne, Timothy B. Smith, and J. Bradley Layton. "Social Relationships and Mortality Risk: A Meta-Analytic Review." *PLoS Medicine* 7, no. 7 (July 2010): e1000316. https://doi.org/10.1371/journal.pmed.1000316.

Huang, Qingyi, Huan Liu, Katsuhiko Suzuki, Sihui Ma, and Chunhong Liu. "Linking What We Eat to Our Mood: A Review of Diet, Dietary Antioxidants, and Depression." *Antioxidants* 8, no. 9 (September 2019): 376. https://doi.org/10.3390/antiox8090376.

Jacobs, Tonya L., Elissa S. Epel, Jue Lin, Elizabeth H. Blackburn, Owen M. Wolkowitz, David A. Bridwell, Anthony P. Zanesco, Stephen R. Aichele, Baljinder K. Sahdra, Katherine A. MacLean, Brandon G. King, Phillip R. Shaver, Erika L. Rosenberg, Emilio Ferrer, B. Alan Wallace, and Clifford D. Saron. "Intensive Meditation Training, Immune Cell Telomerase Activity, and Psychological Mediators." *Psychoneuroendocrinology* 36, no. 5 (June 2011): 664–81. https://doi.org/10.1016/j.psyneuen.2010.09.010.

Janssen, Ian, Valerie Carson, I-Min Lee, Peter T. Katzmarzyk, and Steven N. Blair. "Years of Life Gained Due to Leisure-Time Physical Activity in the US." *American Journal of Preventive Medicine* 44, no. 1 (January 2013): 23–29. https://doi.org/10.1016/j.amepre.2012.09.056.

Katterman, Shawn N., Brighid M. Kleinman, Megan M. Hood, Lisa M. Nackers, and Joyce A. Corsica. "Mindfulness Meditation as an Intervention for Binge Eating, Emotional Eating, and Weight Loss: A Systematic Review." *Eating Behaviors* 15, no. 2 (April 2014): 197–204. https://doi.org/10.1016/j.eatbeh.2014.01.005.

la Cour, Peter, and Marian Petersen. "Effects of Mindfulness Meditation on Chronic Pain: A Randomized Controlled Trial." *Pain Medicine* 14, no. 4 (April 2015): 641–52. https://doi.org/10.1111/pme.12605.

Lauderdale, Diane S., Kristen L. Knutson, Lijing L. Yan, Kiang Liu, and Paul J. Rathouz. "Sleep Duration: How Well Do Self-Reports Reflect Objective Measures? The CARDIA Sleep Study." *Epidemiology* 19, no. 6 (November 2008): 838–45.

Leyva-López, Nayely, Erick P. Gutiérrez-Grijalva, Gabriela Vazquez-Olivo, and J. Basilio Heredia. "Essential Oils of Oregano: Biological Activity beyond Their Antimicrobial Properties." *Molecules* 22, no. 6 (June 2017): 989. https://doi.org/10.3390/molecules22060989.

Lindseth, Glenda, Brian Helland, and Julie Caspers. "The Effects of Dietary Tryptophan on Affective Disorders." *Archives of Psychiatric Nursing* 29, no. 2 (December 2014): 102–7. https://doi.org/10.1016/j.apnu.2014.11.008.

Lo, Yuan-Ting, Yu-Hung Chang, Mark L. Wahlqvist, Han-Bin Huang, and Meei-Shyuan Lee. "Spending on Vegetable and Fruit Consumption Could Reduce All-Cause Mortality among Older Adults." *Nutrition Journal* 11, (December 2012): 113. https://doi.org/10.1186/1475-2891-11-113.

Mayo Clinic Staff. "Aerobic Exercise: Top 10 Reasons to Get Physical." Mayo Clinic. http://www.mayoclinic.com/health/aerobic-exercise/EP00002/NSECTIONGROUP=2.

McCarty, Mark F., James DiNicolantonio, and James O'Keefe. "Capsaicin May Have Important Potential for Promoting Vascular and Metabolic Health." *Open Heart* 2, no. 1 (June 2015): e000262. https://doi.org/10.1136/openhrt-2015-000262.

Mohan, Amit, Ratna Sharma, and Ramesh L. Bijlani. "Effect of Meditation on Stress-Induced Changes in Cognitive Functions." *The Journal of Alternative and Complementary Medicine* 17, no. 3 (March 2011): 207–12. https://doi.org/10.1089/acm.2010.0142.

Moore, Jessy, Michael Yousef, and Evangelia Tsiani. "Anticancer Effects of Rosemary (*Rosmarinus officinalis* L.) Extract and Rosemary Extract Polyphenols." *Nutrients* 8, no. 11 (November 2016): 731.

Murphy, Michael L. M., Denise Janicki-Deverts, and Sheldon Cohen. "Receiving a Hug Is Associated with the Attenuation of Negative Mood that Occurs on Days with Interpersonal Conflict." *PLoS One* 13, no. 10 (October 2018): e0203522. https://doi.org/10.1371/journal.pone.0203522.

Narr, Rachel K., Joseph P. Allen, Joseph S. Tan, and Emily L. Loeb. "Close Friendship Strength and Broader Peer Group Desirability as Differential Predictors of Adult Mental Health." *Child Development* 90, no. 1 (January 2019): 298–313. https://doi.org/10.1111/cdev.12905.

National Center for Health Statistics. "Obesity and Overweight." Centers for Disease Control and Prevention. January 5, 2023. https://www.cdc.gov/nchs/fastats/obesity-overweight.htm.

Newberg, Andrew B., Nancy Wintering, Dharma S. Khalsa, Hannah Roggenkamp, Mark R. Waldman. "Meditation Effects on Cognitive Function and Cerebral Blood Flow in Subjects with Memory Loss: A Preliminary Study." *Journal of Alzheimer's Disease* 20, no. 2 (2010): 517–26. https://doi.org/10.3233/JAD-2010-1391.

Ong, Jason C., Rachel Manber, Zindel Segal, Yinglin Xia, Shauna Shapiro, and James K. Wyatt. "A Randomized Controlled Trial of Mindfulness Meditation for Chronic Insomnia." *Sleep* 37, no. 9 (September 2014): 1553–63. https://doi.org/10.5665/sleep.4010.

Panche, A. N., A. D. Diwan, and S. R. Chandra. "Flavonoids: An Overview." *Journal of Nutritional Science* 5 (December 2016): e47. https://doi.org/10.1017/jns.2016.41.

Prabhakaran, Vijayalakshmi, Thenmozhi Sengodan, and Palaniappan Rajeswari. "The Evaluation of the Virulence Factors of Clinical *Candida* Isolates and the Anti-biofilm Activity of *Elettaria cardamomum* against Multi-drug Resistant *Candida albicans.*" *Current Medical Mycology* 2, no. 2 (June 2016): 8–15.

Ranasinghe, P., R. Jayawardana, P. Galappaththy, G. R. Constantine, N. de Vas Gunawardana, and P. Katulanda. "Efficacy and Safety of 'True' Cinnamon (*Cinnamomum zeylanicum*) as a Pharmaceutical Agent in Diabetes: A Systematic Review and Meta-Analysis." *Diabetic Medicine* 29 (June 2012): 1480–92. https://doi.org/10.1111/j.1464-5491.2012.03718.x.

Ravindran, Jayaraj, Sahdeo Prasad, and Bharat B. Aggarwal. "Curcumin and Cancer Cells: How Many Ways Can Curry Kill Tumor Cells Selectively?" *The AAPS Journal* 11, no. 3: 495–510. https://doi.org/10.1208/s12248-009 -9128-x.

Reynolds, Andrew, Jim Mann, John Cummings, Nicola Winter, Evelyn Mete, and Lisa Te Morenga. "Carbohydrate Quality and Human Health: A Series of Systematic Reviews and Meta-Analyses." *Lancet* 393, no. 10170 (January 2019): 434–45. https://doi.org/10.1016/S0140-6736(18)31809-9.

Salehi, Bahare, Abhay Prakash Mishra, Ila Shukla, Mehdi Sharifi-Rad, María Del Mar Contreras, Antonio Segura-Carretero, Hannane Fathi, Naf-iseh Nasri Nasrabadi, Farzad Kobarfard, and Javad Sharifi-Rad. "Thymol, Thyme, and Other Plant Sources: Health and Potential Uses." *Phytotherapy Research* 32, no. 9 (September 2018): 1688–1706.

Salinas, Joel, Adrienne O'Donnell, Daniel J. Kojis, Matthew P. Pase, Charles DeCarli, Dorene M. Rentz, Lisa F. Berkman, Alexa Beiser, and Sudha Se-shadri. "Association of Social Support with Brain Volume and Cognition." *JAMA Network Open* 4, no. 8 (2021): e2121122. https://doi.org/10.1001 /jamanetworkopen.2021.21122.

Savini, Isabella, Rosaria Arnone, Maria Valeria Catani, and Luciana Avigli-ano. "Origanum Vulgare Induces Apoptosis in Human Colon Cancer Caco2 Cells." *Nutrition and Cancer* 61, no. 3 (2009): 381–89.

Sayon-Orea, Carmen, Maira Bes-Rastrollo, Alfredo Gea, Itziar Zazpe, Fran-cisco J. Basterra-Gortari, and Miguel A. Martinez-Gonzalez. "Reported Fried Food Consumption and the Incidence of Hypertension in a Mediter-ranean Cohort: The SUN (Seguimiento Universidad de Navarra) Project." *British Journal of Nutrition* 112, no. 6 (September 2014): 984–91. https://doi .org/10.1017/S0007114514001755.

Shokri-Mashhadi, Nafiseh, Reza Ghiasvand, Gholamreza Askari, Mitra Hariri, Leila Darvishi, and Mohammad Reza Mofid. "Anti-Oxidative and Anti-Inflammatory Effects of Ginger in Health and Physical Activity: Re-view of Current Evidence." Supplement, *International Journal of Preventative Medicine* 4, no. S1 (April 2013): S36–S42.

Sienkiewicz, Monika, Monika Łysakowska, Marta Pastuszka, Wojciech Bienias, and Edward Kowalczyk. "The Potential of Use Basil and Rosemary Essential Oils as Effective Antibacterial Agents." *Molecules* 18, no. 8 (August 2013): 9334–51.

Smith, Kimberley J., Shannon Gavey, Natalie E. Riddell, Panagiota Kontari, and Christina Victor. "The Association between Loneliness, Social Isolation and Inflammation: A Systematic Review and Meta-Analysis." *Neuroscience & Biobehavioral Reviews* 112 (February 2020): 519–41. https://doi.org/10.1016/j.neubiorev.2020.02.002.

Tang, Yi-Yuan, Qilin Lu, Ming Fan, Yihong Yang, and Michael I. Posner. "Mechanisms of White Matter Changes Induced by Meditation." *Proceedings of the National Academy of Sciences of the United States of America* 109, no. 26 (June 2012): 10570–74. https://doi.org/10.1073/pnas.1207817109.

Twohig-Bennett, Caoimhe, and Andy Jones. "The Health Benefits of the Great Outdoors: A Systematic Review and Meta-Analysis of Greenspace Exposure and Health Outcomes." *Environmental Research* 166 (October 2018): 628–37. https://doi.org/10.1016/j.envres.2018.06.030.

Umberson, Debra, and Jennifer Karas Montez. "Social Relationships and Health: A Flashpoint for Health Policy." Supplement, *Journal of Health Social Behavior* 51, no. S1 (2010): S54–66. https://doi.org/10.1177/0022146510383501.

University of Illinois at Urbana-Champaign. "Dark Honey Has More Illness-Fighting Agents Than Light Honey." *ScienceDaily* (July 1998). https://www.sciencedaily.com/releases/1998/07/980708085352.htm.

Verma, S. K., Vartika Jain, and S. S. Katewa. "Blood Pressure Lowering, Fibrinolysis Enhancing and Antioxidant Activities of Cardamom (*Elettaria Cardamomum*)." *Indian Journal of Biochemistry & Biophysics* 46, no. 6 (December 2009): 503–6.

Xu, Xiaolin, Gita D. Mishra, Julianne Holt-Lunstad, and Mark Jones. "Social Relationship Satisfaction and Accumulation of Chronic Conditions and Multimorbidity: A National Cohort of Australian Women." *General Psychiatry* 36, no. 1 (February 2023): e100925. https://doi.org/10.1136/gpsych-2022-100925.